CLINICAL
COMMUNICATION
SKILLS

CLINICAL
COMMUNICATION
SKILLS

— RICHARD FIELDING —

Hong Kong University Press
香港大學出版社

Hong Kong University Press
139 Pokfulam Road, Hong Kong

ISBN 962 209 371 X

c. 1

HMVK

< F >

Printed in Hong Kong by Nordica Printing Co. Ltd.

Contents

Preface

This book emerged from a growing suspicion that poor clinical communications were causing a great many avoidable problems in health care. Through teaching doctors and nurses communication skills, it was apparent that when these skills were applied substantial changes occurred on a number of levels from individual practice to unit cohesiveness. Teaching communication skills brings about a revolution in the balance of power within the health care industry; a revolution that is long overdue. This book is written for those who need support to bring about these changes. The reader will find information on how communications fit with practice styles, as well as reasons why different recommended styles might be adopted. Some of the material in the early part of the book will provide a grounding in some important theoretical concepts related to clinical communication skills for those less familiar with the area. These introductory sections are by necessity brief and superficial.

This book was conceived primarily as a manual for those involved in training others in communication skills, and secondly as a text for the student. The student will find much in here that is relevant, though the information should not be considered in any way as a substitute for practice. In general, the assumption has been made that the tutor may be relatively inexperienced in training students in communication skills.

The choice of how to organize the text was somewhat difficult. To organize the text along developmental lines, with separate chapters for children, adolescents, adults, the elderly, would raise the question of how to include other special groups. Alternatively, by approaching the subject from a topic orientation, material relevant to different ages and other special groups could be included as and where appropriate. This latter approach was the one eventually adopted.

Given its aims, the text is laid out in what is hopefully a self-evident manner. There are two broad groups of material. The first (Chapters 1 to 4) introduces important background material which tries to provide an outline (or refresher) of issues underlying much of the skills section. Beginning with an introduction to current problems and approaches to overcome these in Chapter 1, Chapter 2 outlines key psychosocial concepts central to communications. Chapter 3 discusses illness behaviour and coping with illness in the self and others. It is important to understand the process of coping and that communication plays a major role in coping. Chapter 4 examines the components of communication and the structure of the interview process.

If Chapters 2 to 4 seem quite lengthy and somewhat discursive, the reader's tolerance is appreciated. A familiarity with the issues discussed in these chapters is important in understanding the reasons for clinical communications. Readers with a background in this area will probably be familiar with much of the material presented in Chapters 2 to 4. For readers who find the material somewhat superficial — again, because the choice of level was not always easy to make — they can omit, after reading Chapter 1, those chapters that cover familiar material and go straight to Chapter 5.

The second section (Chapter 5 to 14) constitutes the bulk of the 'manual' in describing communications components and techniques useful to achieve particular communication goals, beginning with basic skills and proceeding to more difficult aspects of communication. The basics of starting an interview are considered in Chapter 5, where interviewing, asking questions and gathering information are discussed. In Chapter 6, how to guide the interview and how to focus on relevant areas are reviewed.

This is followed in Chapter 7 by the issues and skills involved in handling feelings and emotions in clinical settings, an area many health workers find particularly difficult. Chapter 8 focuses on techniques used in giving information to patients. Specifically, general information about diagnoses, prognoses, treatment and other aspects of care is covered here. The skills and issues involved in handling difficult questions are next explored in Chapter 9, while Chapters 10 and 11 explore more deeply what many consider among the most difficult areas of clinical communications — handling difficult questions and breaking bad news. Chapter 12 considers another difficult area, that of interacting with dying patients and patients in pain, particularly those with cancer.

Chapter 13 changes tack away from patient-oriented communications to consider communications with other health workers and how these can be facilitated.

Each chapter ends with a series of exercises specific to the area of communications under consideration. These exercises are, for the most part, role-play exercises and students are strongly urged to participate and take them seriously. Wherever possible, these role-play exercises should be video-taped for subsequent play-back and discussion. It is unlikely that all the students in a group of 10 can be recorded, so it may be necessary to select one set of students for illustrative purposes. Wherever possible, each student should also have the opportunity for individualized feedback, though this can be done effectively in a group situation. Individual pair training — two students, one tutor — is the ideal if it can be afforded. But throughout this manual, group sizes of 10 to 20 students are assumed to be the norm. Remember, it will ultimately be more efficient to work with several small groups of students than with one or two larger groups. Teaching these skills is labour intensive.

When carrying out the role-play exercises, it is important to have appropriate amounts of space available. Ideally, an interview room or studio with a two-way mirror and microphones for observation and recording should be used if available. In less well-equipped environments, such as a classroom, try to ensure that couples carrying out the role-plays have sufficient room so that they do not interfere with other role-players. Students who demonstrate particularly good performance in certain exercises could be asked to do a live role-play in front of the group (or be recorded for later discussion and feedback).

Tutors should try to design their own role-play exercises which are more congruent with their own particular clinical settings, or to deal with more specific communications problems or tasks. The role-plays provided in this book can only serve as a 'starting pack' and should not be considered adequate for every need, or sufficient in themselves.

Following the exercises, a series of questions is provided to facilitate discussion of the exercises and the skills focused on. Try to raise the thousands of other questions that I have not thought of. Aim to consider not only the technical issues of how to do something, but also the relative advantages and disadvantages of different approaches, the importance of developing an individual style that the student feels comfortable with, and ways to tackle variations in the role-play themes, and particularly the ethics involved in clinical care.

Readers are recommended to work through each section of the manual in sequence, as subsequent exercises build upon and assume a proficiency in earlier skills, as well as providing opportunity for further practice in those same skills. At the same time, they introduce the new material relevant to the current topic.

The format of communication skills described in subsequent chapters represents a combination of different research-lead principles for carrying out a particular function developed by many different workers over many years. There are many ways of doing the things I suggest. The ones described work for me. There are sections that are more controversial than others and there are those that are universally recognized. Thus, these guidelines represent an attempt to develop an empirically based approach to communication skills, but by necessity, the approaches advocated are also flexible. As such it is important to consider them as a set of 'norms' to be followed where feasible. I have tried to develop a consistent style of approach to serve as a model based on first principles which can then be adopted to suit situations I have not considered. These principles are based on mutual involvement, respect and caring for all ages. I hope the importance I place on these principles emerges from the frequent emphasis they receive throughout the book.

Remember, there is no one correct way to communicate, though there are certain times when one approach is likely to be more successful than another. The beauty of communication lies in its almost infinite flexibility. Every individual has his or her own style, and feeling comfortable about what one is doing, even when it is not easy, should be aimed for by both teachers and students.

I am indebted to many people who have in one way or another made this book possible. The people whom I have had the opportunity to work with have helped develop many of my ideas and materials, or encouraged or wrenched me in various directions; they are silent contributors to this book. These include, but are not limited to, John Anderson, Eileen Beeney, Carol Betson, Cheng Yeung Hung, Bob Hobson, Peter Lee, Bea Hung, Irene Matthews, Kerry McCullough, Debra Nestel, Imogen Sharp, Francis Tam and Tony Hedley. Most important are the many people whom, through clinical work, taught me the importance of good communications. My mother, Eleanor Mary Bedingham, who was the first person to teach me about true communications, also must be acknowledged. Finally, I thank my two daughters, Lucy and Brenna, who continue to teach me how much my own communication skills remain in need of development.

Richard Fielding
Hong Kong, February 1995

1

Why Communication Skills?

Introduction

What should a book on clinical communication skills concern itself with? Should the book simply explore the words exchanged between patients and doctors or other health workers about a health problem? That would be inadequate as it excludes the actions and evolution of the consultation. Should a book identify 'bad habits' and offer 'correct' alternatives? It would be possible to break the event down into a number of units and describe or explain their role and sequence in the exchange. However, most units of behaviour are ambiguous in isolation and so add little to an understanding of what happens.

We might view the consultation from a different perspective. What meaning does the exchange have for the participants? Why did they behave the way they did? This may offer a different understanding but lacks clear guidelines to students wanting to improving their communication skill. Yet clearly this level of analysis provides important information to help explain the communication exchange.

This book is about making sense of what happens in communication. To do so, it adopts an approach that incorporates elements of both verbal and non-verbal acts and also tries to examine the deeper principles underpinning clinical communications. These two elements provide the perspective necessary for skills development based on understanding rather than on imperatives.

A research-driven approach to these skills is presented. This emphasizes a definition of communication skill which includes the numerous acts that health workers express in caring for patients. In effect, it defines effective care as a crucial higher-level communication skill dependent on more specific skills like question style and eye-contact.

Philosophical orientation

Underlying the issue of communications in health care is a fundamental philosophy of practice: that patients have the rights to and the needs for information. They may also want active participation in decision making and treatment of their condition as a means of retaining control over their lives. This is based on two key premises: that patients can influence the progress of their illness by their reactions, and that they are the hub of the therapeutic process. Figure 1.1 schematically illustrates the relationship between patient and others. The view that patients have a responsibility for their health should lead to involving patients much more in their own care than is normally the case at present. This change both arises from and facilitates more open communications.

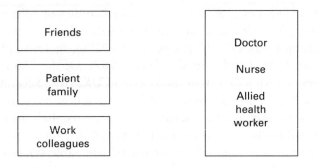

Figure 1.1 Schematic social distance of different groups surrounding the patient.

For some professional groups this threatens established roles and re-sponsibility by spreading these to other professional groups and the patient. Opposition to changes in care reflects unwillingness to provide optimum care if to do so threatens established practice. Yet restrictions on health care spending rely on the adoption of cost-effective means for dealing with disease. It is assumed this will lead patients to be more responsible for their health and more active in negotiating treatment contracts.

State of the art?

The bulk of research on communication abilities of health workers indi-cates a minimal level of skill.

There are a number of problem areas in health care today which can been traced to shortcomings in practitioner-patient communications. The principal areas of medical non-adherence, patient dissatisfaction, failure to detect psychological problems, frustration of staff and intra-staff com-munication are outlined below.

Medical non-adherence

Medical adherence is defined by a number of behaviours, including
1. entering and following a course of treatment
2. conforming to the demands of the treatment (e.g. taking medicines as and when instructed)
3. keeping appointments
4. maintaining behaviour change, e.g. stopping smoking

Medical non-adherence is a problem of epidemic proportions affect-ing between 20% to 80% of all treatment (Ley, 1977; Podell, 1975;

Tebbi et al, 1986). Ley (1977) summarized 68 studies of adherence with a range of medicines, diet, and advice. The median level of non-adherence for all 68 studies was 44.35% (range 8% to 92%). In 1986, the situation was unchanged (Michembaum and Turk, 1987). Of the 750 million new prescriptions issued annually in the USA and UK, over 520 million cases of partial or total non-adherence will be expected every year (Buckalew and Salis, 1986). Among adolescent cancer patients, 40% to 60% fail to take prescribed medication as directed (Tebbi et al, 1986).

Non-adherence is especially poor where detectable symptoms are absent or minimal, and medication is continuously required, for example in mild hypertension (Podell, 1975; Vetter et al, 1985) and diabetes mellitus (Cerkoney and Hart, 1980). There is poor adherence to dietary programmes, high drop-out rates from weight loss programmes, and very poor success rates for smoking control programmes (Sackett, 1976; Becker and Rosenstock, 1984; Meichenbaum and Turk, 1987).

Non-adherence has been attributed to a variety of patient factors including perceived health threats (Lazarus, 1966; Becker and Maiman, 1979), perceived efficacy of prescribed treatment (Becker and Maiman, 1979; Meyer, Leventhal and Gutman, 1985), and conflict between lay and medical beliefs about attributions of disease causality (Fielding, 1987). Most important are consultation factors. Crucially, the behaviour of the health worker plays a critical role in the adherence process. The most influential variables associated with non-adherence include the following (adapted from Turk and Meichembaum, 1987):

- patients' perceptions of the approachability and friendliness of their health worker
- patients' feelings that they are held in esteem and treated with respect
- the degree of patient participation in and understanding of the treatment process
- the degree to which patients feel their expectations are being met
- the amount of supervision by the health worker
- the degree to which the health worker is seen as being considerate of the patient's concerns and feelings
- the degree to which the health worker establishes trust, elicits relevant information, and motivates the patient's cooperation.

The communication skills of practitioners have extensive and sometimes severe shortcomings (Korsch and Negrete, 1972; Byrne and Long, 1976; Ley, 1977; Querido, 1983; Maguire, 1984; OPCS, 1989). They limit not only the ability of the health worker to provide information, but also their abilities to elicit information on patients' key physical problems (Weiner and Nathanson, 1976). This is especially so in the case of psychological complaints (Marks, Goldberg and Hillier, 1979; Querido, 1983).

Information giving by practitioners is also poor, with considerable discrepancies between what patients actually want to know and what the practitioners think their patients want to know. Medical and nursing staff working with dying patients tend to avoid information giving (Maguire, 1984). Reynolds et al (1981) showed that 91% of a sample of cancer patients wanted a diagnosis, 97% desired information about treatment and 88% wanted a prognosis. In Hong Kong, while 68% of dying cancer patients were given a diagnosis, the nature of the disease was revealed only to 20%, and only one in five doctors discussed a prognosis (Fielding et al, 1994). Following myocardial infarction (MI), patients are not given the kind of information they feel they need (Fielding, 1987, 1989); when they are given information they show lower morbidity and consultation rates thereafter.

Patient satisfaction with communications and consultation

When patient satisfaction is low, the patient's evaluation of the consultation is affected (Buller and Buller, 1987). Ley and Spelman (1967) listed five common explanations given by health workers for patients' dissatisfaction with communications:
1. patients don't want to know
2. someone else has told them/will tell them
3. lack of time
4. patient apathy/disinterest
5. reactionary staff attitudes

Even when efforts are made to inform patients, dissatisfactions with communications remain (Ley, 1977).

Dissatisfaction can influence whether or not the patient will return to that practitioner in future or search for a different practitioner — so-called 'doctor-shopping'. Ley (1972) has shown that high rates of dissatisfaction with communication are usually seen together with high rates of satisfaction with other aspects of health care, suggesting that such patients are not general 'complainers'.

Psychological problems

Inadequate communications regarding psychological problems are important for two reasons.

First, psychological problems presenting in the setting of pre-existing physical illness are especially prone to being missed, both by general practitioners (GPs) and hospital physicians. As many as a third of all psychiatric problems are missed, even when the patients are well known to their regular doctor in an out-patient clinic (Querido, 1963; Goldberg and Blackwell, 1970; Maguire, Julier, Hawton and Bancroft, 1974; Brody, 1980; Maguire, Comaroff, Ramsell and Morris-Jones, 1979). Only 17% of cases were detected in one study (Maguire et al, 1979). Only 42% of women with severe psychological upset are identified by the surgeons or GPs caring for them (Maguire et al, 1978). Though most of these studies were carried out over 15 years ago, there has been little improvement since. The detection rate of such psychological problems remains at about 50% (Ormel et al, 1990).

Second, common psychological reactions to physical illness are especially likely to be missed. Many physical diseases generate psychosocial problems for patients (Maguire, 1984a). So do many investigations, treatments and health care procedures that children, adults and the elderly undergo (Mathews and Ridgeway, 1984; Jay, Elliot, Ozolins, Olson and Pruitt, 1985; Anderson, 1987; Martineau, 1989; O'Hara, Ghoneim, Hinrichs, Mehta and Wright, 1989; Viney, Henry, Walker and Crooks, 1989; Fielding, 1991). More serious diseases, such as cancer, cause many psychological problems for patients (Brinkley, 1983; Maguire, 1984a; Derogatis, 1986b).

It is not just life-threatening diseases that generate problems for patients. Almost all patients are affected psychologically by disease; the less that they know about the disease, the more it is likely to upset them, particularly if the symptoms are highly visible or interfere significantly with normal activities (Thorne, 1993).

Frustration and demoralization of staff and alienation of patients

Health workers frequently encounter frustration and demoralization arising from poor communication.

Medical and, to a lesser extent, nursing education focuses primarily on a cure-oriented approach with the patient viewed as a biomechanical organism. This has resulted in 'disease care', the predominant style of Western (allopathic) education and health care delivery. This biomechanistic model overlooks the fact that *care* constitutes the basis of health care. Professional education needs to emphasize communication skills to a greater degree. Only in the last 10 years have communication skills become a part of medical, nursing and paramedical curricula, though the need has been widely recognized for decades (Simpson et al, 1991).

To staff trained in cure-oriented biomedicine, dying represents a failure of the 'hospitals-make-us-well-again' philosophy. When physicians and nurses avoid dealing with patients' emotional and other psychological needs, they are defeating their own best efforts. The management of the patient becomes more difficult. Often cure is not possible, nor is control of the disease. Most health professionals acknowledge that many patients die in hospitals. But death represents a failure of the biomedical ethos. Staff don't enjoy facing frequent reminders that the biomedical model usually doesn't succeed, unlike a garage that mends broken motor cars.

Lack of open communication between staff and patients also unnecessarily restricts the roles of the doctor and nurse. Often there is frustration and dissatisfaction at the lack of opportunity to provide more personalized care, or to contribute to and participate in decision making about individual practice. Changing the style of care can help reduce some frustration but is likely to emphasize limitations of existing communications.

Multidisciplinary team communications

Research indicates communication failures are extensive between health care teams and their members. Consequences include failure to keep other team members informed, duplication of expensive tests, failure to detect, acknowledge or take action on positive test results and persisting with discontinued procedures (Massey and Reimels, 1986; Tsunematsu, 1988).

These failures often arise from the belief that it is unnecessary to keep other staff informed of decisions made by physicians (Massey and Reimels, 1986; Tsunematsu, 1988). Familiar justifications are offered: insufficient time or belief that other parties knew and were taking action.

How have these problems come about? Several reasons seem to be important.

First, awareness of the communications needs of patients has been relatively slow to filter through to health workers. Research began about 40 years ago, with most information appearing since the 1970s. Many senior health workers influencing policy and practice were trained more than 10 to 15 years ago. They did not have the benefit of this knowledge. Many such health workers are role models for junior staff. Most medical and paramedical training programmes even today fail to give adequate time to teaching communication skills. Nursing degree programmes tend to be a slight exception.

This is partly because health workers, particularly doctors, assume no particular skills are required to communicate with patients. Even if special skills were needed, it was, and often still is, believed that the apprenticeship education method still predominant in training health professionals leads to the acquisition of communication skill by osmosis. Unfortunately, the opposite happens. Doctors at least become less effective and sensitive communicators with increasing medical training (Alroy, Ber and Kramer, 1984).

Third, both patients and health workers have made greater demands for more information and participation in treatment-related decision making (Angell, 1984). Health workers are becoming increasingly aware that present practices are unsatisfactory and that many workers lack the skills needed to deal with many areas of practice.

Fourth, awareness of the influence of psychosocial factors in the onset, reaction to and recovery from disease and illness is greater. Stress (Mason, 1968; Lazarus, 1966), heart disease (Fielding, 1991), cancer (Burgess, Morris and Pettingale, 1988; Ramirez et al, 1989), recovery from surgery (Skipper, Leonard and Rhyme, 1978; Mathews and Ridgeway, 1984), susceptibility to infectious diseases (McKeown 1976; Totman and Kiff, 1979; Kiecolt-Glaser et al, 1986) and many other areas demonstrate the intimacy that exists between social environment, behaviour and health.

While environmental limitations are frequent explanations for poor communication, they all too often become excuses for poor skill. In most cases, adequate time and staff are available. The true problem is one of priorities. Tasks have historically taken precedence over people in health care settings, and talking with patients is still likely to be perceived as laziness rather than delivering care.

Implications

Health care communication skills involve merging knowledge gained from research into perception, memory, cognition and learning, with social skills. Social skills are social interaction skills involving conversational or verbal skills and the recognition and expression of non-verbal cues. Most people are well experienced in these areas. But because they use these skills every day does not mean that they are competent in those skills. Some people are highly skilled while others are significantly handicapped socially because of inadequate social skills.

Most health workers can hold a conversation, ask questions and undergo an interview, with varying levels of skill and confidence. However, most of us benefit from practice in these areas. Moreover, health workers must communicate effectively with people from a variety of social and cultural backgrounds about complex topics. For many health workers, situations arise daily which require sensitivity and a high degree of communication skill. It is important that they be skilled in communication. Many, sadly, are not.

Learning and teaching communication skills

This section considers different approaches to teaching clinical communication skills, and what happens to the practice of health workers who are trained in such skills. If you are a student using this book as a textbook, you may want to skip parts of this section, specifically those parts focusing on different approaches to training. However, you are recommended to read the sections on effects of practice and on the use of this book. But the only way to effectively learn any skill is to practise it. In other words, you should rehearse these skills in role-play situations with a friend or colleague as an important stage in learning before trying them with patients. Ask the friend for feedback on how you did. Talk about your feelings. Try to find a style that feels comfortable and right for you.

If you are using this book as a training manual for teaching others, this chapter is important. It contains information on optimizing the teaching of communication skills and should be read before later sections.

Benefits for health workers

We all believe we know how to communicate, don't we? Many health care students believe communication skills training to be unnecessary, communications being 'common sense'. If that is true there is a tremendous lack of common sense in our health care systems today.

Communications training involves skills learning in which two things must happen. First, learning a skill requires practice and feedback. You must try to do it yourself rather than listen to someone tell you how to do it, although that is an important preliminary step. Second, practice is crucial to improve performance.

Research shows that with effective communication skills training, people are better communicators, becoming more sensitive to those features of interactions that are important. This increases satisfaction with interactions both for health care consumers and workers and in turn with the service available. Moreover, effective communication skills among health workers will facilitate communications even with patients who are themselves poor communicators. Good questioning skills can help obtain better information from a patient who is a poor communicator (Brown, Weston and Stewart, 1989). A health worker with good interview skills can often make a better diagnosis, provide more appropriate treatment, and effect greater change in patient behaviour. Good exposition (information giving) improves recall, increases patient satisfaction and treatment adherence, thus making more efficient use of scarce resources. Improved treatment efficacy and reduced wastage benefit both the health care system and the individual.

Methods for skills training

Giving constructive criticism and encouragement about people's performance will more effectively enable them to modify their performance in future. Structured communications-oriented training programmes are increasingly taught in medical schools for example. Most try to teach a range of basic skills to students. These include increasing students' awareness of the patients' experience of hospitalization (e.g. Carmel and Bernstein, 1986), avoiding the use of jargon (e.g. Scott and Weiner, 1984), and specific interview styles (e.g. Wells, Benson and Hoff, 1985). Some programmes focus on increasing satisfaction with consultations (Evans, Kiellerup, Stanley, Burrows and Sweet, 1987).

Despite these efforts, shortcomings remain. Many programmes do not evaluate their effectiveness. Other programmes offer only limited training in basic interviewing skills. But the problem remains one of priorities. Task learning or factual study continues to take precedence over communication skills.

1. Trial and error

Most health workers learned their communication skills through trial and error. Despite this, many have excellent skills. Others do not. In health care, trial and error is usually highly inappropriate. Where communications are concerned, the consequences of errors may not be very apparent. Even when they are, the origins are usually attributed to 'difficult patients' rather than the interviewer.

Leaving nurses, doctors and allied health workers to learn skills by trial and error has not generally been successful. Individual health workers who become model communicators are the exception rather than the rule. Indeed, though there are some gifted health communicators, the vast majority of us are not. Relying on trial and error may generate a lot of avoidable problems for both the patient and worker while learning proceeds, and thereafter if inappropriate skills are learned.

2. Apprenticeship schemes

Apprenticeship programmes are established and tried means of imparting technical and professional knowledge; students are expected to integrate their own skill with the example of their peers or role models. Unfortunately, poor communication skills among role models simply pass on bad habits. Also the student may not easily separate good communication behaviour seen in others from behaviours which reduce effective communications. As we have already seen in the previous section, the problems and complaints expressed about current skills leave little room for doubt that current role models have flaws. Instructors are either not teaching the correct skills in a way that students are able to learn, or they are not teaching the correct skills because they themselves don't possess them.

3. Individual versus small group learning

Specific communication skills training is therefore needed. Choosing individual or small group approaches to communication skills learning comes down to resources. If five can be trained to the same level it takes to train one in about the same time, there is little advantage to individualized training. Individual training using dyadic one-to-one student-patient followed by video feedback is preferred by some, but is costly in terms of time and resources. Small groups are adequate as audio-visual technology can provide additional instruction and feedback. Small group teaching enables students to work independently and yet cooperatively in a team. This is how health care is delivered. Groups also provide a safe supportive social framework within which to explore roles and behaviours during learning. Both have obvious advantages for learning and developing expertise in communication skills.

The final size of a group depends to some extent on the availability of time and the range of support resources, such as video systems. As a teacher, it is important at the beginning of each new group to establish relationships with and between the students. Students who are strangers may find some of the activities difficult at first. Chapter 2 contains several exercises in self-awareness, which can be used to familiarize a new group. Where time is limited, getting the group 'up and running' effectively as soon as possible is important. Frequent discussion of the activities and experiences of the group, and their feelings are valuable; they can also be threatening, and should be introduced with sensitivity. The interested reader should consult texts on teaching within small group settings and the techniques available to facilitate group function.

4. Modelling and the use of video

Modelling occurs when we observe the consequences of other people's (the actors') behaviour and then subsequently adopt that behaviour ourselves. Modelling is a highly effective means for learning certain types of knowledge, particularly social behaviour and can be used in several different ways to teach communication skills.

First, illustrating an idealized approach to a particular social interaction, where the model demonstrates how to interview a patient, for example. The students observe, and then try the skill themselves. A second approach, not strictly modelling, is to use the 'worst' approach or 'spot the problem' demonstrations and to ask students to identify particular problems or errors made by the role model, and/or to suggest alternative approaches to different parts of the filmed exchange. This can then be followed by the 'best' approach — the modelled behaviour.

There are many video tape programmes available for teaching specific aspects of communication skills — for example on how to break bad news — produced by different universities in the UK, Australia and the USA. These tapes can provide a model of how to act under given circumstances to achieve the best result, but they may not always be professionally or culturally appropriate. They provide models of skilled experts we can copy. It is recommended that this type of education videotape be used to stimulate discussion of the appropriateness of behaviour and the effectiveness of certain approaches. Commercial tapes may also be useful.

Video technology also provides an ideal form of feedback for students, particularly when accompanied by expert commentary on performance. Videotaping an interview between a student and a 'patient' provides clear illustration to the students of their performance. Repeated use leads to finer and finer improvement in communication skills.

Effective use of video technology is indispensable in communication skills teaching. At least one camera, videotape recorder and video monitor are essential equipment for skills training and should be used for demonstrations and feedback. Training can be done without video, but where possible, every effort should be made to utilize it in teaching. In circumstances where video is not available, or where sheer numbers make individual use impractical, an observer can make detailed notes of performance for later discussion with the student.

2

Basic Psychological Processes in Communication

Introduction

Communication is based on cultural, social and psychological systems. These are very influential. For example, social rules for turn taking in conversation are strong. So, frequently speaking out of turn interferes with smooth conversation and brings censure. Likewise, many psychological processes are involved in communication. Two are of key importance: perception and memory. Some of the features of perception, particularly social perception, and memory relevant to clinical communications are discussed in this chapter.

What is communication?

> A human being is not a box with one orifice for emitting chunks of stuff called 'communication', and another orifice for receiving it. And at the same time, communication is not simply the sum of the 'bits' of information which pass between two people in a given space of time.
>
> Birdwhistell (1970)

The word communication and the word common come from the same linguistic root, implying 'a connecting passage or channel', the means whereby something is transferred from one place to another. In human communication it is messages that are transferred.

Messages contain information. Senders of messages intend certain meanings. Receivers of these messages almost always ascribe meaning to messages. Meaning is imposed upon a message as much by the listener (or reader) as by the speaker (or writer). This is an important point. The intended meaning and the imposed meaning may differ considerably. We tend to think most information exchanged between people is transmitted by language. But much information is carried by non-linguistic aspects of communication such as posture, 'body-language', and context, than by words and phrases. Words do not by themselves determine meaning.

Moreover, people do not simply respond to words and movements but to what they are interpreted as meaning. It is the imposed meaning that we respond to rather than the specific verbal message (which, without all of the accompanying cues, becomes largely meaningless).

The intent to communicate particular meanings is important. What is fascinating is that the intended meaning is so often understood by the listener. Consider a spoken conversation. The meaning perceived in a message is dependent upon a wide array of interlocking factors. These include the message content, which is influenced by the nature of the message. This in turn is influenced by the context of the message, not only in terms of preceding and subsequent information, but also its congruence with other levels of concurrent information. The sender of the message, its timing and purpose, all affect the message's context.

The message has important implications for the receiver-sender relationship, and for the expectations, current concerns and past experience of the receiver. These implications in turn influence the nature of the response, and so on. This tiny, highly simplified fragment reflects only basic processes in a conversation. Some conversations used in health care (e.g. psychotherapy) include the whole spectrum of two or more people interacting over time (Hobson, 1984). This is a much more complete view (see Bateson 1973 and Birdwhistell 1970 for fuller accounts).

To summarize, human communication involves the production, selection, sifting and evaluation of different levels of simultaneously presented information (verbal, situational, relationship, visual, etc). From this, the overall meaning is derived. This, in turn, is modified by antecedent and consequential influences. The result is an exchange of meaning. People interpret messages using a vast array of cues. When these cues are absent, altered or unfamiliar — as they may be for patients in an hospital environment — the chances of misunderstanding increase drastically.

But how do we decide which information in the environment is part of a message? And how do we sort out the the message from everything else? To answer these questions, we need to consider some of the psychological processes involved.

Psychological processes relevant to communication

By necessity, discussion of psychological processes here is very cursory and superficial. The interested reader should consult specialist texts on the particular topic in question.

Perceptual processes

The selective nature of attention

The continuous assault of sensory information that is always present would swamp us if we could not select out information. Selective attention acts like a kind of searchlight which we can move over the range of sensory information available, mostly at will. The attention process is an active control process (Keele and Neale, 1978), determining what is attended to and how information is processed. It sets itself to expect certain inputs and inhibits and distorts unwanted or conflicting information.

Imagine you are at home with a painful tooth abscess. The telephone rings. It is a dear friend from whom you have not heard for many months ringing to arrange for a visit. You are very pleased to receive the call and eagerly exchange news with your friend. After the conversation ends, you hang up the phone. Then you notice you were unaware of your aching tooth, and that, on thinking about it, the pain has re-emerged as before. Imagine waiting in a dentist's surgery for your check up. You hear a scream from the room next door. How do you react? Do you look in the direction from which the scream originated? Would you feel nervous or alarmed?

The first example illustrates how switches in attention can quickly exclude irrelevant information. The second example illustrates how the relevance of a stimulus can attract our attention unwillingly. However, were we not able to select an input, we would be unable to function socially at all. Some people with damage to the anterior cerebral cortex experience profound attentional deficits, making normal social interaction almost impossible. For these people, all incoming information is given equal priority with no opportunity to select items requiring response. Any meaningful response then becomes extraordinarily difficult.

Perception, not seeing

Perception is the process of organizing our sensory field in such a way that meaning emerges. This purposefully suggests that meaning is an emergent property of the perceptual process and not some disembodied stuff contained in a message. This is a *crucial* point. Perception is more than just seeing or hearing. The retina responds only to light intensity and frequency, the cochlea only to air pressure changes, the nociceptor (so-called 'pain receptor') only to mechanical distortion or heat. Yet instead of experiencing light or dark, silence or noise, pressure or heat, we perceive a world, hear speech and birdsong and 'feel' pain.

Sensory features, such as lines or shades are perceived as object characteristics, such as colour, shape and size, and not as independent stimuli. This act of perceiving complex stimuli results in the emergent experience of objects. Increasing familiarity with common stimulus configurations leads to assumptions about the objective world. Thus, the appearance of a wound is informative to an experienced health worker, but not to a student.

The perceptual system has a number of relevant features:

(a) **Perceptual stability.**   This is the tendency for features of our sensory field, such as size and shape, to be perceived as constant. We are not born with this ability but acquire it within the first six months of life. Awareness of the self as separate develops about the same time as our sense of the autonomous existence of objects, and the two are probably closely related (Richards, 1974). Constancy phenomena occur in all modes of perception, not just in the visual system. We do not make judgements solely on the basis of new information, but combine this with knowledge from past experience about similar events to produce a hybrid interpretation. Experience with a symptom, for example, is therefore a vital part of establishing what it means.

(b) **Stimulus organization and perception.**   The way that objects, rather than object characteristics, are perceived implies that perception 'organizes' incoming sensory information into a form which has potential meaning within the framework of the perceiver's current concerns. An illustration of this in health care is how a set of apparently unrelated signs and symptoms come to be perceived as a disease.

Knowledge of stimulus organization tells us that the perceptual system relies on rules for interpreting percepts. These rules are often relied on more than the sensory information itself. The perceptual system searches for patterns, sometimes creating them where they do not exist. An example is a doctor interpreting a set of signs as confirming a diagnosis (which may be incorrect). Pain is a further example. Vague sensations perceived by patients are more likely to be interpreted as pain following diagnosis of cancer compared to before the diagnosis was disclosed (Turk and Fernandez, 1989).

The perceptual system seems to search for the best fit of incoming sensory information with pre-existing templates of experiential information. Psychologists sometimes call these templates schemas (Cohen, Eysenk and LeVoi, 1986).

(c) **Context and experience.**   What determines the 'best' interpretation of an ambiguous stimulus such as a symptom? Symptoms fall into what are called fuzzy categories. Fuzzy categories are ill-defined or uncertain representations characterized by a number of optional properties. The uncertainty in fuzzy categories can be resolved by looking at when the symptom occurs. With past experience, this helps to clarify the meaning of a symptom. Context is crucially important in perception as it helps resolve uncertainty or ambiguity.

A range of different contextual cues can be identified. Some are intrinsic to the situation (e.g. adjacent regions in a scene) (Frisby, 1986), while other contextual cues are more general, such as conversational aims — social, lecture, warning, etc. (Bateson, 1972). Context provides a higher level of information about the nature of the stimulus. Familiarity with the same or similar stimuli on previous occasions provides a probability estimate for interpreting the present stimuli. This phenomenon is thought to be very important in diagnosing infrequently occurring diseases (Kahneman, Slovic and Tversky 1982). Stimuli that occur frequently are more expected than those which occur infrequently. Therefore, it is likely that commonly occurring interpretations are more likely because they are more common. However, this is not always the case.

Most important in terms of communications are social and cultural contexts. Social contexts are the social settings within which different communications occur. It is quite possible to have a conversation with a complete stranger on the other side of the planet via Internet; though both persons may be alone with their respective computers, there is still a social context within which they communicate. Cultural contexts are the prevailing norms and values of a social group which have profound influences over the range of human behaviour within that social group. These norms and values dictate the circumstances in which behaviour can be acceptably displayed. For example, while crying is something that all people are capable of, there are quite strict rules, display rules, which determine where, when and by whom crying is acceptable. Within these contexts, crying acquires different meanings — as indicating sadness, joy, fear, depression, loss, beauty, exhilaration, despondency — which are then attributed as *causes* of the behaviour. In this way, crying acquires a signalling role controlled by the context. A person feeling the need to cry may exercise restraint until an acceptable context is present. In this manner, the context controls the behaviour. The context may also be a cue for the behaviour, for example a funeral in southern European cultures will feature much florid crying among certain individuals of whom the behaviour is expected. The absence of (expected) crying also acquires attributed meanings.

Why are these issues important here? Selective attention, stimulus organization and context, together with past experience, are processes which can influence what is attended to and its ascribed meaning. In later chapters these phenomena are all used to improve communications.

Social perception in health care

The perception of people is especially important in health care as it influences how we behave towards each other. This in turn influences how and what we communicate.

People not only change their appearance and behaviour, but also possess invisible features such as character and attitudes. Because people present such a wide range of stimuli, we tend to rely on both learned

social perceptions of behaviour and habits that reduce sensory information overload. These are discussed below.

Roles and stereotypes in health care

Roles are obligatory patterns of behaviour expected in certain circumstances. For example, doctors are expected to help the sick, to be
responsible and not act to harm life. When Acquired Immune Deficiency
Syndrome (AIDS) was first identified, some nurses in San Francisco refused to nurse AIDS patients; no obstetrician could be found to care
for a woman carrier of Human Immune Deficiency (HIV) virus in a
New Dehli hospital. Both nurses and doctors were violating role prescriptions. We all have many roles, some of which we are required to
enact concurrently. A woman is expected to be a wife, mother and doctor,
for example. Other combinations of roles are considered incompatible,
such as a doctor becoming a patient's lover. Roles help us to predict
the behaviour of others and to determine our own behaviour. Thus, they
reduce uncertainty. Role violations are often penalized out of proportion
to the gravity of the violation probably because they threaten social
predictability.

By comparison, stereotypes are simplifying classifications, usually of
people and social situations, based on a few features, and much belief.
They involve no prescriptive component. Examples of stereotypes are
those of the complaining elderly and the reckless youth. Individuals may
be evaluated in total, on the basis of such superficial features as age, race,
creed, occupation and gender. Generalizations, such as stereotypes, are
not really true beyond a limited set of instances from which they are
derived, and many may not be based on fact at all. The pre-judging of
people on the basis of stereotypes leads us to perceive others in a certain
way (prejudice). This may become a problem when we change our behaviour towards others on the basis of stereotypes, and when such changed
behaviour results in discrimination (Bar-Tal, Graumann, Kruglanski and
Stroebe, 1989). Stereotypes of homosexuals contributed towards discrimination against AIDS patients by religious groups and many staff in USA
health care facilities during the early 1980s (Black, 1986). Stereotypes are
important in setting up expectations among staff and patients about the
nature and intentions of others.

Stereotypes then are over-generalized beliefs over-applied to all members of a group. The rare occurrence of people who fit the stereotype is
taken by most of us as proof of the stereotype's accuracy, despite their
rarity. This reflects people's tendency to seek confirming evidence and
reject contradictory evidence for a proposition (Roth and Frisby, 1986).
For example, new data gathered in an interview seems to be used by

health workers to confirm first impressions, rather than alter them (Johnson, Kurtz, Tomlinson and Howe, 1986).

Both stereotypes and roles are used by people to evaluate others. Hence stereotypes held by health professionals influence communications and relationships with patients. Doctors tend to spend more time per interview with patients who possess middle-class speech characteristics compared to those possessing working class speech characteristics (Buchan and Richardson, 1973; Cartwright and O'Brien, 1978).

Clinical decision making is similarly affected. Social factors, such as social class, economic background, ethnicity, gender, physical appearance, and family influence affect clinical decision making (Eisenberg, 1978). Patients designated as 'lower class' are more likely to be given graver psychiatric diagnoses and poorer prognoses, than patients of other social classes when the only difference between the two groups was designated social class (Trachtman, 1971). Poorly educated elderly people and those of lower social class seem more likely to be diagnosed as dementing (O'Connor, Pollitt, Treasure, Brook and Reiss, 1989). Women are more than twice as likely to be diagnosed as obese, even though obesity is more prevalent among men than women (Franks, Culpepper and Dickinson, 1982). Johnson et al (1986) reported that student health professionals rated the most preferred trait in a patient as 'attractive', and the least preferred as 'a whining tone of voice'. The most desirable patient in this study of both male and female health students was a young, attractive, white, middle-class woman, and in spite of the fact that this patient was a poor and inconsistent history-giver, the characteristics most frequently used to describe her were 'reliable source of information' and 'open and honest'. It is not socially acceptable to admit that attractiveness influences perception, whereas it is more acceptable to admit that 'openness and honesty' do (Johnson et al, 1986). Attractive but difficult patients are more likely to be rated as good patients, even when they are not, than are unattractive patients, even when they are good patients, especially if little is known about the person (Eagly, Ashmore, Makhijani and Longo, 1991).

In explaining the 'open and honest' influences, Johnson et al (1986) assume that health workers are aware of their bias, but choose to hide it. However, it may also be that health workers are not continually aware of their bias. This seems much more likely, especially in the areas of perceived social competence and adjustment (Eagly et al, 1991).

In summary, perception is an active process relying for the large part on habits and probabilities to simplify information load and processing. These habits lead us sometimes to see things that are not there and at other times miss those that are there. There are many examples of misdiagnoses, often discovered too late. For example, a week after being informed that corrective surgery for a separate congenital condition could not be performed, a 25-year-old man who was emotional, distressed and complaining of severe unilateral head pain was diagnosed by his physician as having migraine brought on by the stress of disappointment. The patient died one week later from systemic shock and cerebral abscess. The tendency of the perceptual system to prefer confirmatory over contradictory information is something that all health workers should beware.

Memory in health care

Memory is important in health care communications for at least two reasons:
* patients need to give autobiographical information to health workers
* patients need to retain information given to them by health workers

Memory has for many years been considered as having two categories: long-term memory which retains information for long periods of time, and working or short-term memory, a scratch-pad type of store or processor for retaining information that is being worked on. More recently, up to nine 'memory' systems have been proposed (Teasdale and Barnard, 1993). Other features of the central nervous system influencing information processing include structural limits on the processing of serial information (such as speech or music), and the conscious processing of only one modal input at a time (Teasdale and Barnard, 1993). The mode refers to the nature of information. For example, we cannot read text and listen to a conversation simultaneously and process both inputs unless we switch back and forth from input to input. Both require the language processing capacity of the brain (the morphono-lexical subsystem), but only one can use it at any one time. So, only one or the other input will be accessed and subsequently processed and recorded or memorized. However, we can process different information modes, such as pictures and speech simultaneously because different cognitive subsystems appear to be involved. Some people are skilled at integrating simultaneously presented aural and visual information, for example when singing a musical score during a concert.

Short-term memory processes important aspects of the environment. Our limited attentional ability restricts short-term memory. This places limits on how much information patients will recall from what they are told. Most patients can only retain about seven units of information at any one time. More information simply overwrites the earlier information, which is then lost.

Secondary, or long-term, memory is the main memory store, with virtually unlimited capacity and potentially lifelong duration of storage.

Yet not all information that is stored in long-term memory can be re-trieved after many years, weeks or sometimes just minutes.

Autobiographical memory

Of particular importance to health workers is the patients' memory of per-sonal events, that is, their history. Remembering what has happened to you is different from remembering what you know about algebra or history.

One aspect of memory focuses on objective reality — the world (Tulving, 1972). The more frequently an objective event occurs, the better the general knowledge that comprises it is recalled. **Semantic memory** stores information on the basis of its meaning for the person. This, in turn, derives from the general cognitive (mental) structures that a person develops over many years. On the other hand, events that happen to people are stored episodically. **Episodic memory** relies on the coding of information attributes from personally experienced unique episodes, which may be more superficially processed (Herriot, 1974). Episodic memory focuses on the self. The more similar events occur, the more difficult they are to differentiate from each other. General characteristics of the events are recalled, but differences tend not to be. This last point is important when interviewing patients with long-standing conditions, for whom it becomes increasingly difficult to recall individual symptom events.

Flashbulb memory is a term given to infrequent but vivid and detailed recollections that people have of important events (Brown and Kulik, 1982). The events resulting in flashbulb memories usually have high emo-tional content for the individual. The nature of these memories remains controversial. An example might be seen in victims of disasters or war, where they have witnessed killings or severe injury to themselves or oth-ers. This often results in Post-Traumatic Stress Disorder among survivors, which is characterized by vivid, intrusive memories of the event(s).

Long-term memory for skilled task performance along with other 'recording' systems may also exist but do not concern this topic.

Influences on memory

How do memory systems perform and what affects their performance? Before we can get information out of memory, we must ensure that information goes into memory and is retrievable. As we all know, forget-ting can be a major problem. Forgetting may reflect a decayed memory, but inability to find the information among a vast memory field is more likely. This in turn may reflect encoding failure. This is losing something because you fail to note where you put it, rather than it moving from its place or because it has deteriorated.

How information is processed (encoded) influences how well it is stored. When trying to memorize facts for an exam, recall is much better if the material is understood (that is, if it has meaning). Names and dates are more difficult to recall than the events associated with them. This reflects deep versus superficial encoding. Information which has greater meaning for a person is said to be more deeply encoded and thus better stored (Craik and Lockhart, 1972). Elaboration of information and identification of meaning most effectively benefits recall. In contrast, the volume of information can be reduced by simplifying the information.

Thus, patients' retention of information can be improved by making it more meaningful. Organization of information into meaningful categories may be used to enhance the recall of greater blocks of information.

Context provides a powerful aid to memory. Information encoded in a given context (physical environment, emotional environment, social setting, etc.) may be less effectively recalled in a different context. Police investigators jog the memory of witnesses by taking them to the scene of the crime, or by re-enacting the crime in its setting.

New information can interfere with information already memorized (retroactive interference), and material already memorized can interfere with newly learned material (proactive interference). This may lead to confusion. Furthermore, the position of a piece of information in a sequence also affects recall.

Individuals have their own strategies for learning or memorizing information. These may be simple or complex and may help to make the information more meaningful. Furthermore, we make inferences and interpretations of information during processing which effects what is encoded. Such inferences may be encoded simultaneously or even instead of the original information, giving highly idiosyncratic memories for events and information in some circumstances.

Herriot (1974) has emphasized the difference between the encoding that occurs at the presentation of verbal material (which would be in terms of discovered meaning) and the decoding that occurs at recall (which would be in terms of constructing messages from meaning). This can result in a phenomenon known as creative memory. In creative memory, repeated minor changes can occur to a piece of information as it is stored and recalled, resulting in the evolution of the memory into some inaccurate form. So it is important to remember that memories may not reflect the information that was initially encoded. Individual interpretations and idiosyncratic encoding strategies mean that verbatim recall of verbally presented material rarely occurs. It is the meaning material has for the individual that appears to determine what is recalled.

Self-awareness

Identifying and acknowledging your own feelings can sometimes be difficult. We might feel a mixture of things, unsure of what we are feeling exactly, or unable to name it. We may fail to understand why we feel that way. It may not always be necessary to know why we feel a certain way, but it is important to acknowledge our feelings.

How do you become more aware of the information your own feelings can give you? Self-awareness is an ongoing process throughout our lives. In communicating, our own thoughts and feelings come partly from our current concerns. Perceptions contribute to the exchanges that occur between people. The social demands of situations help generate these. In other words, we should be aware first and foremost that we are highly responsive products of our social and psychological environments. People are created by a complex, lifelong interplay between current thoughts and feelings built on past experience and social environments. These generate expectations of how the physical and social world functions. These expectations affect how we respond to events.

Two important personal dimensions exert powerful influence on how a person behaves. These are self-esteem and self-efficacy. Self-esteem refers to the view we have of our own worth. In a thesaurus, esteem is synonymous with regard, respect, confidence, reputation, to cherish, and to love. Self-esteem is how you apply these values to yourself. Where self-esteem is low, this can have a significant effect on both what and how you communicate with others, and how you respond to others' communications and behaviour to yourself.

Self-efficacy cognitions are the attitudes, beliefs and perceptions we have of our abilities in relation to interactions with the rest of the world. They include how much we believe in what we do, in our abilities to accomplish the things we view as important, how we attribute cause and effect in relation to the things we value, and how effectively we can cope with demands (Bandura, 1986).

Self-esteem and self-efficacy are closely related. Indeed, self-esteem may be said to arise from appraisals of self-worth interacting with other self-efficacy beliefs.

Summary

Attention powerfully affects the meaning of messages, which messages are attended to and whether information contained in the message is attended to or not. This may seem like a long winded way of saying that when people don't listen, they don't remember what is said to them. It is. But it is more than this. It also tells us how stereotypes and roles, for example, set up expectations and attitudes which we then seek to confirm through our selective attention to affirming features. An example is that female patients are generally believed to be more 'neurotic', when in fact there is no evidence to support this view.

A range of contextual and expectancy factors affect the meaning of the information used to make decision about patients. These kinds of influences need to be considered in relation to how people experience illness and their coping responses to ill-health. Perceptual effects are central to the coping process. Again, as we shall see, communications are of central importance in the understanding and facilitation (or inhibition) of the coping process during illness.

Exercises in self-awareness

The following exercises explore self-awareness and make some suggestions for using your own feelings as information on the state of communications. Most of them are in the form of experiential work that you can explore on your own.

Recall when you last felt anxious, afraid, unusually happy or sad. In each situation, there was almost certainly some expectation by you of some kind of outcome, or expectation by others of some kind of behaviour by you. How these expectations affect you is intimately dependent on self-efficacy beliefs. Expectations bring with them the possibility of being fulfilled or not, and perhaps perceptions of success or failure. Self-esteem is often increased by perceived success and decreased by perceived failure.

These reactions have considerable influences on interactions with others and an awareness of the view you have of yourself; beliefs about your abilities, and the nature of the world can effect important changes in your social behaviour.

There is a strong chance that other events unrelated to the experience might have been seen in a different light. If you were anxious other people probably detected your anxiety. Your anxiety was probably not just a 'feeling', but more a state. Your thoughts were anxious thoughts, your posture was an 'anxious' posture, your face wore an 'anxious' expression, and your behaviour was characteristically 'anxious'. Do you experience anxiety particularly in one or two aspects of yourself, or does it seem to manifest itself in all the different dimensions of you?

You may not experience anxiety, but the same applies to other feeling states. You may be very skilled at not revealing your feelings, in which case it may be more difficult for others to identify what you are feeling. Some people are so effective at not revealing their feelings that they are not even evident to themselves.

The following exercises are designed to help you to become more aware of your feelings. Simply reading through them will not provide much benefit. However, if you make an attempt to spend some time to repeat and work on these exercises, they can provide a starting point for widening your awareness. What you will get out of these exercises in terms of greater awareness will be proportional to the time you spend getting to know yourself better.

1. Try a small experiment. Take a few moments and think of a time in your life when you were anxious or frightened about some significant event or person. Allow your face to take on the expression of an anxious person and clench your fists and your jaw muscles. Keep thinking of this event. Was it threatening? Were you scared?

    Think about how the event feels now. Are you anxious now, or do you feel other feelings?, If you feel anxious, is it real anxiety, or just a memory? In what way are the two different? It can be difficult to distinguish the two, except for the intensity and the spontaneity of the 'real' anxiety. If you imagine the situation as vividly as you can, some of the feeling associated with that event will come back. Working the other way around, do you find it is possible to recall similar situations more easily when you feel in a particular mood? Pleasant situations when you feel happy, unhappy situations when you feel sad, and so on. This is more likely to happen with the recall of sad event than happy events.

2. Keep thinking about that event. Did it change the way that you related to other people? If it did, in what ways? For how long?

3. Moving on from this, try to recall several events from your life that you consider significant and try to regenerate the feelings that were associated with them. Are you able to re-create the event, and how does doing so make you feel now? Are the feelings still strong, or are they different? In what way are they different and in what way are they the same?

4. Can you locate the feelings physically inside of you (or outside)? If so, whereabouts? Are they actual sensations, such as an increased heart rate or 'butterflies' in the stomach, or are they more vague and indistinct?

5. Focus on one event that still evokes strong feeling in you. Think about what that event was. Now think about what it was about the event or its meaning to you that lead you to feel the way you do now. Was it the event itself, or some consequence or implication of the event? If so, what? Try to follow this line of thought to see if you can better understand the components of your feelings that might relate to different parts of the event and its consequences.

6. Do the following exercise somewhere you will not be disturbed when you can devote about 15 minutes to it. Keep your eyes closed over the course of the exercise. Try to become aware of as many sounds as you can. Make a mental list of them. Keep going over the different sounds until you have them all. Next, note the sensations there are in different parts of your body: feet, legs, buttocks, arms, back front, inside abdomen, inside thorax, shoulders, neck, face, mouth, head. Spend some time exploring these sensations.

7. This exercise can be done in a group, or with a second person. There are certain expectations of social behaviour that are deeply ingrained in some cultures, such as maintenance of eye-contact during a conversation. Explain to your partner the purpose of the exercise. Sit facing your partner and look at your partner's eyes. Try to maintain eye-contact for as long as possible. At the same time try to remain aware of how you feel. Think about why you feel that way. What do these feelings say to you?

    Alternatively — with someone who is a good friend and would not be easily upset by unusual behaviour — keep looking at your friend even if your friend is looking at you. Notice how you feel. What are the feelings?

3

Illness Behaviour and Coping With Illness

Educational Objectives

By the end of this chapter, you should be able to

- differentiate between illness, disease and sickness
- define illness behaviour and offer examples
- discuss how family and cultural structure affect the construction of illness in adults and children
- list the roles adopted by individuals in a family coping with illness
- discuss factors affecting the meaning of illness
- discuss how illness meaning affects the patient experience
- define coping
- differentiate between emotion-focused coping and problem-focused coping
- recognize the need for patients to make sense of illness events within their own world view
- describe the association between patient coping and beliefs about cause of illness
- describe how developmental level affects coping ability
- give reasons why children should be actively involved in communications and their care
- list factors which help or hinder successful coping in ill children
- list common strategies used in different developmental stages to cope with the demands of illness
- recognize adaptive and maladaptive forms of coping

Introduction

This chapter has two goals. First, it gives information about how different age groups cope with illness. Second, the content provides important evidence in favour of adopting a higher priority for communications and psychosocial care in health care delivery. Two key concepts underlie the material covered and link it to subsequent chapters.

1. Strategies which increase the sense of mastery of patients and relatives over the adaptive demands of illness are important to successful coping. Conversely, actions generating helplessness-passivity tend to be linked to maladaptive coping.
2. Communication is important in assisting adaptive coping. Material is presented emphasizing: (a) information gathering to assist coping; (b) maintenance of open and effective communications channels; (c) the development of key relationships.

Health workers can help maximize patient/family information resources, teach practical management skills, and encourage self-mastery during illness. Giving patients information and encouraging participation in care are therapeutically important. Information is power. It adds to personal resources, enhances accurate appraisal and optimal coping, and makes adaptation and recovery more likely. Thus, communication becomes therapeutic. Withholding information encourages dependency and is as unethical as withholding beneficial treatment.

Illness behaviour

When we are unwell, we might wait, take an aspirin, see a doctor, or cry in pain. Mechanic (1962) used the term illness behaviour to help explain 'the ways in which given symptoms may be differentially perceived, evaluated and acted (or not acted) upon by different kinds of persons'. So illness behaviour is what people do when they believe themselves to be unwell. Sickness is that which interferes with a person's ability to fulfill his or her social roles, and is the result of being defined by others as unhealthy (Twaddle, 1981).

We learn our beliefs, attitudes and behaviours about illness primarily from the family. These are passed on to the next generation by example (Mikail and von Baeyer, 1990), social reinforcement of approved behaviour, and by ignoring or disapproving unacceptable behaviour. These cultural influences shape our responses to events and people and the beliefs we hold about ourselves in relation to our environment: perceptions of control, powerfulness, self-efficacy and other aspects of our lives.

We learn our roles and we also learn what we can expect from others. For example, repeatedly placing females in subordinate caretaking roles helps significantly shape the views held by both sexes of the roles, status and power of women in a society.

The meaning of illness

Illness (unwellness as opposed to disease) is a social construction. We are considered ill because people agree about what is and is not accepted as illness. Illness is a symbol for forms of discomfort which the person has learned to attribute to changes in the body. Disturbances originating outside the body, for example a difficult personal relationship, may also be experienced in terms of bodily disturbances. Often illness is identified in adults and children when it interferes with their ability to carry out activities. In children three to four years old, something counts as an illness if it interferes with the child's relationships with significant others and is labeled as illness (Wilkinson, 1988). The gatekeepers who label states as illnesses are parents, our kin system, and the medical profession (Friedman, 1970), who serve as the final verifiers.

People from the same sub-cultural backgrounds tend to share both a common vocabulary and common expectations about the causes and responses to illness. This may more likely lead to consultation than if patients are from a different culture or sub-culture to the health worker (Friedson, 1961).

Culture and gender

Correspondingly, attitudes towards maintaining health, responses to illness, and roles during illness and sickness differ between social groups. The multi-cultural nature of most urban societies means that a wide diversity of beliefs and behaviours regarding health and illness is seen in allopathic health care systems. A health worker in a large metropolitan area will care for people from many ethnic and cultural backgrounds. Hence, there is a strong need to be sensitive to differences in illness behaviour and health care practices.

A failure to recognize that different cultures construct illness in different ways leads to a kind of cultural arrogance: that only Western models of illness and Western-style treatments are acceptable. Being closed to different sub-cultural models of illness impairs practitioner-patient relations considerably.

Key Points

Different ways of constructing illness result in different perceptions of what is important causally and therapeutically. Exploration
of these by asking the patient about what they think is happening
to them is important to help establish a common language for
defining, representing, discussing and ultimately solving the problem.

Gender differences are an important cultural issue in health care. The
majority of medical staff are males and the majority of nursing staff and
paramedical professionals are female. It has been repeatedly observed that
these professional roles reflect dominant gender roles within society. Within
the family, mothers more than fathers carry out care of the sick, but
fathers may be more involved in accident treatment. Wilkinson (1988)
describes this as reflecting the care versus cure roles of females and males
in many societies, including the health care industry. Common gender
problems faced in health care include cultural barriers to Asian women
undergoing pelvic examination, especially by a male physician, or being
cared for by a male nurse. Male midwives are rare for these reasons. This
raises questions about women consulting male doctors (or nurses) and
male patients with female doctors (or nurses). Do you prefer to see a male
or female doctor? Why? Combinations of gender and cultural differences
compound communications difficulties between professionals (see Chapter 13).

This introduction has raised several complex issues that are beyond
the focus of this particular book. Though not considered further here,
they are important contextually, influencing the effectiveness of clinical
communication skills.

Coping with illness in the self

Illness and consulting

Illnesses are events, sometimes accompanied by pathological changes in
the body or behaviour. Illness almost always arises from the broad context of a person's life. This is true of a common cold, lung cancer,
'schizophrenia' or diabetes. But these conditions — perhaps with the
exception of schizophrenia — all have partially understood pathologies;
they are all currently recognized diseases. Sometimes people are ill yet not

visibly diseased. They may consult a doctor because problems in coping with life make them feel uncomfortable in some way.

Conversely, some people have very clear and marked pathological changes but they do not experience that sense of being unwell called illness. These people are diseased but they are not ill. Some people carry on with their lives even with serious symptoms. Sometimes the person's ability to understand their health status is affected. Neuro-degenerative diseases including Alzhiemer's, Pick's, Creutzfeld-Jakob, multi-infarct and atherosclerotic dementias have this effect. Other problems, such as 'schizophrenia', can impair a person's ability to make effective judgements about behaviour.

Whether or not there is a clear pathology, ill individuals will, by definition, change their behaviour. For most health workers in hospitals and clinics, contact with the more seriously sick and incurable is the rule. Yet for every patient that is seen in hospital, there are ten in the community; for every symptom displayed by a patient, many more are not seen by health workers. These phenomena are called the 'illness-iceberg' and 'symptom-iceberg' respectively.

So, most ill people, signs and symptoms never reach a doctor or hospital. People with symptoms follow broadly similar courses of action. Most symptoms and illnesses are minor, self-limiting conditions which people often recognize having had before. They pose no threat. They improve no matter what the patient does, so any treatment may seem 'effective'. They may be ignored or self medicated with over-the-counter drugs.

Most extended and extended-nuclear families are able to cope with minor illness by a slight redistribution of responsibilities and roles where necessary. Single people and single-parent families encounter more difficulties. Few single parents can afford the luxury of having a rest or easing up on their routine responsibilities if they feel ill.

If symptoms are persistent or unusual, but not severe enough to interfere with daily activities, there is a waiting period during which the symptoms are monitored by the patient (Nerenz and Leventhal, 1983). During this time, the sufferer might talk with a network of non-professionals, friends or relatives, about the symptoms and possible responses; this is called the lay-referral system (Friedman, 1970). During this time, the person decides on the meaning of the experience in terms of cultural and personal constructs. If the meaning of the symptoms are construed as an important or potential risk to health, a doctor is then likely to be consulted.

Research suggests experiential aspects of illness, such as symptoms, need to match more abstract aspects such as name, nature, prognosis, and so forth. When discrepancies exist between different aspects of the illness experience (e.g. symptoms in the absence of a detectable diagnosis, or treatment in the absence of perceived symptoms), people attempt to resolve the discrepancy (Nerenz and Leventhal, 1983). This might happen by seeking further consultations, a change in symptoms, rejecting a diagnosis (Fielding, Wong and Ong,1992) or reducing adherence to treatment.

Friedman (1970) proposed that a person who lives 'in a society where medical defined illness and impairment are extraordinarily common will, because they are accustomed to them, report fewer symptoms of illness than would a medical examiner'. Conversely, this implies that in an almost symptom-free community, new ways of expressing illness might be expected to manifest once traditional diseases all but disappear. (See for example post-viral syndrome or chronic fatigue syndrome (Ray, 1991).) What roles might 'new' illnesses serve for patients and health workers?

Coping

Coping is the process of adapting to demands for change. Lazarus and Launier (1978) defined coping as 'effects, both action-oriented and intrapsychic to manage (i.e. master, tolerate, reduce, minimize) environmental and internal demands and conflicts among them, which tax or exceed a person's resources' (p. 311). How successful we are depends partly on our beliefs about ourselves, on our past experience with similar types of events, and on the accessible resources available. We must also be motivated to cope. That is, we must want to overcome the demands inherent in adapting to changed circumstances.

Key Points

It is important to remember that coping is a *process*, and not a state. Unfortunately, the bulk of research on coping has failed to consider this important point, with the result that much published research is contradictory or unequivocal.

Coping research has developed several theoretical positions which appear consistent. These models fall into two broad groups. Established models focus on accepting or rejecting the threat inherent in demands for change. Popular examples are the psychoanalytic defenses, such as projection, repression, reaction formation, and so forth. More recent formulations include acceptance-denial (e.g. Cassem and Hackett, 1971; Havik and

Maeland, 1986; Levine et al, 1987). Monitoring-blunting is conceptually similar (Miller, 1987) but describes information gathering styles adopted under demanding situations. This model proposes that some people seek more information by becoming more alert within their environment, while others do the opposite. The parallel to the acceptance-denial dichotomy is not difficult to see.

A second group of coping models conceptualize coping from a functional perspective. Under these models, successful coping alters demanding circumstances in some manner that minimises or avoids the impact of threat. This has been called instrumental or problem-focused coping (Folkman and Lazarus, 1980) or danger control (Nerenz and Leventhal, 1983). Instrumental coping can be thought of as active coping. Conversely, a person can ignore circumstantial aspects of the problem, trying instead to control any emotional disruption arising from the problem or its accompanying threat. This is called emotion-focused coping (Folkman and Lazarus, 1980), and may be thought of as a more passive form of coping.

Adaptive coping in illness seems to be related to the patient's perceptions of the event as a chance event or not. If the illness is seen as a chance event, the patient is more likely to adopt a passive emotion control coping (Parkes, 1984). Where the perceived threat to the patient is high and their coping resources perceived as low, or poorly developed, maladaptive coping may appear, presenting in a variety of ways. If the illness is perceived as controllable, patients may seek to increase their control over the illness and their resources (instrumental coping). This may include searching for information, a desire to participate in decision-making about the illness and treatment, and so on.

Where coping is unsuccessful or perceived resources are so poor that extreme threat is anticipated by the patient, a number of pathological coping responses may materialize. They include panic-driven desire to escape, paranoid features, and aggressive and even violent behaviour (see the case history of Stan, Chapter 8).

Less extreme failures to cope may result in patients experiencing depressive reactions characterized by vegetative disturbances such as loss of appetite, loss of interest in activities, frequent crying, feelings of sadness, depressed mood, loss of motivation, loss of interest in sex and low self-esteem. Depressive reactions are particularly common when the patients risk losing something valued or perceive themselves to be helpless to influence the event (Maguire, 1984b).

A number of studies have explored these dimensions of coping in illness and consistent findings support the validity of the dichotomous models. The problem is that these models do not easily allow us to see how the *process* of adaptation develops over time.

Using a qualitative approach to explore coping has produced some interesting insights into how these somewhat static models might fit together. In a small study by the author on 34 patients admitted to a hospital in Australia for acute myocardial infarction (AMI), a structured interview was completed at 24, 48 and 72 hours after admission. The purpose was to explore how coping strategies evolved over the immediate period following the AMI. How patients perceived their circumstances was clearly important. Whether patients adopted a realistic view of their circumstances, accepted or rejected responsibility for what had happened to them, what meaning the AMI had for the patients, and whether they had active or passive attitudes to instrumental coping were commonly demonstrated dimensions to the patients' coping.

When AMI was not perceived as a chance event, patients more often demonstrated the following: saw the AMI in more positive terms; accepted some responsibility for the AMI; held realistic views of their circumstances; tried to make sense of the event in their own conceptual framework; desired more involvement in treatment decisions; desired to control or modify perceived risk factors; and desired more health knowledge to apply to future prevention. Many of these responses are instrumental in that they reflect attempts to increase control over their illness.

These patients clearly attempted to make sense of the event by repeatedly examining their situation and events leading up to it. It was important for many of the patients to understand why this illness had happened to them. Many patients were frightened and felt a strong need to 'protect' themselves from being emotionally overwhelmed by the threat in what had happened to them. This is similar to selective avoidance (Perlin and Schooler, 1978), or suppression (Parkes, 1984), rather than denial of reality, which is supposedly a blanket blocking out of the reality of the situation, reputedly very widespread in patients following AMI.

The following extract illustrates this point.

Pt:*   . . . (It) seems like it didn't really happen, couldn't have really happened. I remember it all so clearly, but keep on thinking 'Did it really happen?', but I've got paddle-marks on my chest, so it must have happened. You know, kinda couldn't sink in, and . . . it seems to be that's the way it is when you have something really big happen. You go into some kind of shock thing where you don't bridge or reach the problem. Maybe that's a good thing 'cos I don't know if I really forced it . . . I don't know how I would take it.

* Pt: Patient,   HW: Health worker.

I consciously make an effort not to constantly dwell on it. I think if I allowed myself to, I would. At the moment, y'know, because it's all new and uhm . . . , yeah, I find it hard not to. When people come to visit me I talk about anything except what they want to hear, and that's 'How are you?'

HW: How does that help?

Pt: It creates a bit of balance I think, for me. Whereas if I got really emotionally upset, that may not be good for me physically. At the moment I don't feel I want to go that far with it. But I want to be supported. If I know I'm supported, I'll feel OK and even that's supporting me by keeping myself in balance a little bit, perhaps by thinking 'No, don't think about it now, leave it'.

HW: Is it important to keep your emotions under control right now?

Pt: It's not important; I'm just too scared not too.

Note how only parts of the event have been selectively avoided. Others have reported this as an important positive coping mechanism (Vaillant, 1976; Parkes, 1984). This periodic peeking at the experience seems to serve the purpose of desensitizing the patient to what has happened. In this controlled way, over at least the three days following the AMI, the patient gradually increased the amount of exposure given to the event and its implications. In this fashion, the patient retained control over emotional responses while becoming familiar with and making sense of the experiences. The last statement in the above example indicates how, what at first glance appears to be, an emotion-control strategy also serves instrumental purposes as well, and *vice versa*.

A belief by patients that they can do something about their problem is an important determinant of effective adaptation to the changes accompanying illness. With information, support and guidance, patients are motivated to adapt to the demands presented by illness. In this way, new approaches to dealing with problems can be explored and a greater sense of mastery over the problems arises. Successful coping is constructive adaptation to the demands brought about by illness in such a way that the patients and their family can continue to function in a positive and creative fashion.

Coping and developmental level

A young child lacking the experience and skills of an older child or adult is forced to use more basic or primitive coping responses to deal with change. As a child ages, a wider range of skills and resources become available, until as an adult, an extensive range of coping responses are potentially available. For example, Bande (1990) reports diabetic children aged less than 12 years cope by trying to actively control instrumental factors. After 12 years of age, however, in addition to instrumental coping, more effort is spent on adapting to living with the disease.

Throughout the child's younger years, parental intervention supplements the resources available to a child. But change is inherent throughout our lives and events like the birth of a sibling, mother returning to work, going to school for the first time, all contribute demands for coping on the child. Through the successful solution of these adaptive demands, the growing child builds not only a repertoire of skills, but growing confidence in the ability to cope with change. The very experience of learning to cope is a growth-enhancing part of life.

Key Points

The nature of an illness event and the time of its onset will determine the coping demands made on a person. The developmental level of a person in terms of coping may not resemble the person's chronological age.

Coping is influenced by the developmental stage of the person. A child may cope with demanding change by demonstrating a loss of control over behaviour or body. School performance may deteriorate, a previously passive child may become aggressive or uncooperative. A previously toilet-trained child may begin to soil or become enuretic at night. An older child may show other socially disapproved behaviour such as pilfering or truancy. Adults often classify such behaviour as 'bad' or naughty, but in most cases they reflect the child's inability to cope effectively with the demands for change.

Regressive coping is where a person at a particular developmental level resorts to coping strategies more consistent with an earlier developmental stage. It is common for people of all ages to adopt regressive coping strategies if they feel unable to succeed with more mature strategies. Some people fail to adopt mature strategies at all, relying on primitive coping throughout their lives.

More primitive coping strategies when seen among older children, adolescents or adults tend to be classified, often unjustly, as pathological reactions, yet they may simply reflect people using methods they know best. These are explored in more detail below.

Coping among children and adolescents with illness

The dependence of the child on the family means that the child's coping with illness must be seen in the context of its family. The meaning of a child's illness affects its own response (Willis, Elliot and Jay, 1982) as well as the parent's response to it. Children from about the age of three onward have the capacity to distinguish between health and illness. As they get older they formulate their own ideas about the causes and meanings of what others have called illnesses. But children's low status within society may mean that their opinions are never consulted (Hart-Zeldin, Kalnins, Pollack and Love, 1990).

In our paternalistic system, children are given the message that while they may not have been responsible for what is happening to them, they also have nothing to contribute to becoming well. This attitude is widespread despite children preferring involvement and being quite able to care for themselves, especially if given clear guidelines about what to do (Lewis and Lewis, 1990). The child not only has the unwillingness of the health care professions to overcome but also parents who may feel their role is being undermined if they abdicate care to the child.

These attitudes do not help children develop responsibility and hence a sense of powerfulness in the face of illness. A family attitude that the causes of disease are beyond the control of people can have the same effect. Blaxter (1983) describes certain attitudes to illness in a sample of working class women who believed that for many illnesses there was an inevitability arising from lifestyle. This was especially so where poverty was concerned. For many of these women, disease was something that ran in families. One was born vulnerable and that giving in to illness was a moral weakness. By blaming factors that were external to the person, such as 'germs', culpability could be avoided. These and other parental attitudes set the context for children's learning about health and illness.

Children's beliefs about illness

In infants, illness can disrupt the bonding process between the mother and child. Sick neonates may not develop early social turn-taking with the mother. Their cries may be more ambiguous leading to an impaired relationship between the mother and child. Premature neonates are less likely to respond appropriately and are more likely to be victims of later child abuse (Wilkinson, 1988). In the context of marital discord, mothers are more likely to experience puerperal depression (Cox, Conner and Kendell, 1982), which interferes with maternal communication responses to their infant (Wilkinson,1988). This can profoundly affect later communication competence, social relationships and possibly later intellectual deficits in the child (Coghill, Caplan, Alexandra, Robson and Kumar, 1986).

Bibace and Walsh (1980) reported nursery school children believe illness to be inherent in certain objects or persons and that proximity to these lead to illness. In older children, the authors identified a 'contamination' view of illness causality, which gradually became more sophisticated to about 11 years of age. The presence of 'germs' was adequate cause in the minds of those under 10 years but older children developed more complex multi-causal descriptions of illness.

By the time children reach secondary school age, they appear to be trying to integrate educational ideas of bodily function with concepts such as sleep, nutrition and, presumably their predominant family attitudes (Wilkinson, 1988). They have integrated ideas and attitudes about causality, responsibility and treatment.

Adaptive and maladaptive adjustment

Successful adjustment to illness among children is found in families in which there is '(a) a clear separation of the generations; (b) a satisfying of each other's emotional and psychological needs; (c) flexibility within roles; (d) toleration [sic] for the individual; (e) communication which is direct and consistent, and tends to confirm the self-esteem of others' (Shapiro, 1983).

Adaptive patient responses reportedly include 'realistic self-reliance acceptance of physical limitations but with the development of compensatory activities; being able to express sad, angry or anxious feelings; guarded optimism during periods of clinical quiescence; denial and isolation of affect to cope with emotional distress; a focus on the here and now; and the effective use of support individuals' (Shapiro, 1983). Other important influences on positive coping include independence, peer contact, school participation and achievement and participation in other activities normal in childhood (Shapiro, 1983).

In addition to coping factors, there are other factors which seem to be protective in that, when present, the demand experienced by the child is minimized, or coping resources are maximized. Rutter (1979) identifies several mediating features of the child's psychosocial environment which seem to offer some protection against stressful demand, such as illness. These are favourable home environment, self-esteem, the availability of environmental options, structure and control within the family, and stable relationships with adults.

Maladaptive coping responses in children have been anecdotally described rather than based on empirical data. Based on this, Shapiro (1983) identified the prolonged poor adjustment as characterized by fearfulness, inactivity and dependency. Alternative patterns associated with poor adaptation seem to include being overly independent, engaging in prohibited risk-taking behaviours, or demonstrating resentful, hostile attitudes to non-disabled or other persons. In the pre-adolescent, maladaptive responses often manifest themselves in the form of behavioural and psychological disturbances, including demoralization, self-denigration, denial and depression. These are consequential on attempts to cope with the stressful demands in normal activities of daily living (Shapiro, 1983).

Secondary gain and increased attention occur, though these can be counter-productive in the long run. They rarely offset the depression, anger, fear, social isolation, shame, sense of deviance, passivity, over-dependence, and hyper-sensitivity that are common in the chronically ill child.

Families can compound or interfere with children's attempts to cope successfully. Family attitudes associated with impaired family coping include severe and unchanging denial of the reality of the illness, hypochondriasis in other family members, and unresolved anger directed at other family members with no effort at resolution (Shapiro, 1983). These are likely to inhibit coping in the child. The illness itself is often less menacing to the child than the familial response to the illness (Gutton, 1978).

Because of the integration of the child within the family unit, malfunction of the family can increase illness in the child (Miller, Court, Walton and Knox, 1960), and raise consultation rates for minor illnesses (Christine-Seely, 1981).

Adaptation to chronic conditions, such as diabetes mellitus, has been argued to have at least three phases (Laron, Galatzer, Amir, Gil and Karp, 1989). First a shock phase where there may be a tendency to reject the diagnosis and seek a second opinion. This is followed by a phase involving adaptation to the demands of the treatment regimen. Finally, adaptation to the chronicity of the condition needs to occur if adjustment and normal development is to follow.

Anxiety is commonly experienced in children coming into contact with health care. In older children, anxiety about medical procedures and hospitalization is dealt with in a variety of ways. A mixture of active and passive coping behaviours similar to those described among adults are seen (Broome, Bates, Lillis and McGahee, 1990). Active coping is associated with lower levels of reported discomfort and pain than is passive coping (Broome et al, 1990). A similar picture is seen among adults (Egbert et al, 1964), reflecting the benefits of perceived control.

Hospitalized pre-school children most frequently cope by information seeking (watching and visual examination) and instrumental action (tension reduction involving self, control by active participation, and control by preventing or delaying an event) (Ritchie, Caty and Ellerton, 1988).

Acutely ill children appear to use fewer coping behaviours in high stress than low stress situations compared to chronically ill children (Richie et al, 1988).

A major problem arising from chronic illness in adolescents is social isolation. Dealing with issues of personal identity is a major developmental task of adolescence and is disrupted in illness. The chronically ill adolescent may need to maintain dependence on parents while resenting the maintenance of a child-like state. Low self-esteem and self-doubt are common. There may be conflict over the giving and receiving of parental care. If financial or marital problems exist, the child may feel a burden on the family. Communications between the caretakers and adolescent may deteriorate drastically (Waechter, 1987).

Facilitating children's coping with illness

For children, illness has been described as coping with a series of demands caused by loss (La Montagne, 1987; Wilkinson, 1988): loss of wellness, loss of freedom to play, loss of important social events, loss of functions, and in severe illness, loss of family and life. Adults facilitate children's coping and peers facilitate older children's coping by improving resource appraisal and controlling the perception of threat. La Montagne (1987) proposes 21 coping interventions for use with children. Of these, 10 involve information or communications, while the remainder focus on developing self-responsibility and environmental supports.

Coping with illness in family members

Healthy family coping has not been widely studied. Part of the problem is whether the family can be said to cope as a unit, or whether the coping is merely an aggregate of the strategies of the individual family members. However, Shapiro (1983) lists the goals of family coping as follows:
1. having a sufficiently large adaptive capacity to accommodate the changes caused by the illness
2. maintaining a sense of membership in the family for the ill person
3. reorganizing the family and assigned roles
4. re-establishing an emotional baseline and the mastery of resentful, self-accusatory and other negative feelings
5. maintaining relationships which afford some gratification and at the same time fulfill its members' physical and psychological needs.

Most research on family coping has relied on stage models and focused on severe or life-threatening illness. However, stage models offer no explanations, are of limited validity and place restrictions on the range of possible individual responses. There is no reason to suspect that a demand-resource model of stress would not be as appropriate for a family unit as it is for an individual. It is also possible to identify instrumental strategies and strategies aimed at minimizing family disruption (the group equivalent of emotion control?) akin to those used by individuals. Therefore, these conceptualizations for individual stress and coping will be applied to the family unit in this chapter.

How the family copes is influenced by the past illness coping style of the family, the success of such coping, and the quality of the relationships within the family. These in turn are affected by the family's contacts with the outside world, such as employment status, income and extended family and other social networks.

Coping with a child's illness

A variety of primary responses have been described in response to confirmation of serious illness, including shock or rejection of the initial diagnosis, attempts to seek a second opinion or to shop for other treatments (Wilkinson, 1988; Lo et al, 1994). Individual reactions including anger, guilt, anxiety and depression have been reported (Shapiro, 1983).

Identifiable problem-solving strategies in families include information-seeking actions (designed to increase family resources and more accurately appraise the threat presented by the illness); identifying and procuring the best treatment available (or affordable); and intentional self-help strategies, including relaxation, dietary regimens and religious activities aimed at modifying the illness. Responses designed to limit the impact of the illness on the family include cognitive strategies such as positive thinking, engaging in more family interaction aimed at increasing pleasant activities for the affected child or family as a whole, and activities designed to minimize the emotional impact of the illness on the parents, the ill child, and any siblings.

Family coping with minor illness

Most traditional families accommodate minor illness in children without too many problems. An ill child may demand more time and contact with the mother, impairing normal parental activities. (While the mother may not be the principal caretaker, this has been assumed to be the case. Hereafter the main caretaker will be referred to as the mother.) Maternal reactions to her child's illnesses have been reported in several studies to be the major determinant of the child's recovery (Skipper and Leonard, 1978;

Wilkinson, 1988). The mother is also the main etiological factor in subsequent behavioural disturbance in the child (Shapiro, 1983). Finally, maternal behaviour is reportedly of major importance in consultation behaviour (Shapiro, 1983), demands for medication (Howie and Bigg, 1980), and possibly hospitalization (Maclure and Stewart, 1984; Reed, 1990). Some marital discord between parents is expected (Shapiro, 1983) and there is a risk of siblings exhibiting behavioural disturbances.

Family coping in chronic illness

In chronic illness the increased demands on the individuals within the family can effectively reduce its buffering capacity. Even where a child was mistakenly diagnosed as having a chronic illness, and the mistake rectified afterwards, the parents continued to perceive the (well) child as vulnerable years later (Carey, 1969).

Parental responses are varied. Research has rarely studied adaptive responses, but by extrapolating from research on individuals and coping, adaptive instrumental responses likely include the following: increased information-seeking; exploration of new strategies to achieve everyday tasks and meet needs; successful redistribution of roles within the family to accommodate changes due to the illness; adopting responses which facilitate the child's control over life; discouraging dependency while promoting independence; maintaining open and honest communication within the family; maintaining close and supportive family relationships which do not distort the balance of attention in favour of, or away from the sick child; and maintaining active social contacts and activities. Additional adaptive responses facilitating emotion-control include: dealing effectively with anxiety; maintaining an optimistic view of the future; focusing on the child's positive characteristics instead of the limitations caused by the illness; maintaining a sense of competence within the family; developing or maintaining spouse communications about feelings; taking regular breaks from the domestic environment; and dealing effectively with feelings of guilt.

Five categories of coping identified among 30 families of children with cancer were: experiencing the disease as challenge, as probation, as misfortune, as fate, and as punishment (Peterman and Bode, 1986). Thorne (1993) has described the process of families developing confidence to manage both the disease *and* the health care system to obtain adequate care.

Maladaptive family coping

There is growing information about maladaptive coping of families, mostly of children with chronic illness. Common maladaptive responses reported include various forms of denial or refusal to accept the diagnosis, followed by high levels of guilt, helplessness and passivity among parents (Valman, 1981). Over-protectiveness, unrealistically low expectations of the child, and the encouragement of dependency (Strand, 1979) and chronic grief or sorrow (Fraley, 1990) occur. Marital function, parental sleep, appetite and coping with external demands (e.g. employment) may be compromised (Shapiro, 1983). Finally, rejection, criticism, or over-involvement with the ill child to the exclusion of other family members, distorting family activity and finances in the direction of overcompensating for the illness have been reported (Shapiro, 1983). The ill child in families who are not coping well may be hospitalized more frequently for more minor reasons (Reed, 1990).

Sibling's reactions to illness in a brother or sister are also more powerfully influenced by the reactions of the family than the illness (Taylor, 1980). Siblings concurrently experiencing other demands, who have poor relationships with other family members, few outside friends or support systems and limited communication skills seem to suffer the most behavioural disturbances (Shapiro, 1983). They may experience feelings of jealousy toward the ill child who is receiving increased attention (Lademann, 1980) while they feel deprived of parental attention. Guilt commonly results from believing the illness may have arisen from the sibling's ambivalent feelings (Rothstein, 1980). They may develop physical symptoms, behaviour disturbances, and sleep problems including nightmares and enuresis (Shapiro, 1983).

Supportive interventions can minimize sibling reactions to severe or chronic paediatric illness. Support groups have been used successfully in the USA to facilitate exchanges of feeling and sharing of experiences in siblings of cancer sufferers (Heiney, Goon-Johnson, Ettinger and Ettinger, 1990). Communication with and education of parents about consequences for siblings is urged to minimize sibling disturbances (Thorne, 1993).

Illness in parents of children

Where six-month to four-year-old children are separated from their caretaker by the *parent's* admission to hospital, bonding is seldom disrupted in traditional families. In single parent families, foster care of the child may contribute to later relationship problems with the parent. Prolonged illness in parents can affect children if it interferes with the normal pattern of parent-child activities (Wilkinson, 1988). When this happens, the pre-adolescent child tends to acknowledge illness in the parent. The child's response is affected by his or her developmental level, the presence or absence of siblings and their age. Older adolescent siblings can help considerably in the practical running of a household, but the demands to cope with additional responsibilities at a premature age can place a child under substantial stress.

Up to the time of writing only one study was found in the literature which examined the effects of maternal illness on the family (Lewis, Woods, Hough and Bensley, 1989). The number of illness demands the father experienced was a significant predictor of his level of depression. This affected marital adjustment as did the wife's type of disease. Both illness demands and level of marital adjustment significantly predicted the type of coping behaviour the family used. More frequent illness demands and higher levels of marital adjustment were associated with familial introspection (coping behaviour characterized by frequent feedback, reflection, and discussion in the family). The quality of the father-child relationship was significantly affected by this type of coping behaviour. Introspective families had fathers who reported more frequent interchange with their children.

Illness in the parents of adults

So far the focus has been on illness and coping among children. More often it is elderly adults who are ill, and relatives will likely be adult children of the ill elderly. Where these relatives have their own families, a buffering and supportive network is available to help cope. In the nuclear family, the physical separation of the family from the ill elderly probably minimizes disruption among vulnerable family members, such as children. In most societies, it is women who provide care of the sick within families, including elderly family members (Jones and Vetter, 1984). Women also provide the bulk of care to the terminally ill living in the community (Cartwright, Hockey and Anderson, 1979).

Because adults have available to them a wider array of coping responses, they are often assumed to be able to deal adequately with illness in elderly parents. However, this assumption often helps isolate carers of the ill elderly. Carers report certain problems of care, such as incontinence as particularly stressful. Almost one woman in five caring for an ill relative reported 'almost unbearable' levels of stress, with daughters reporting more stress than spouses (Jones and Vetter, 1984). Hence, because the caretakers are adults, it should not be assumed that they will be able to cope effectively with the demands of caring for a sick parent, a relative, or even a child. This may be even less likely, paradoxically, where the caretaker has a family of his or her own. Under these circumstances, the caretaker may have a greater number of demands from the family as well as from the elderly parent. From this, it can be predicted that supportive families are more beneficial than non-supportive families of caretakers.

Summary

Coping is facilitated by close supportive and positive communication of caring and information to enable greater control over perceived threats. These communications are in turn dependent on good relationships with both close others and, by extrapolation, with health workers, who should provide the bulk of information resources.

Exercises

1. If you were sick, who in your immediate family would take care of you? If the main breadwinner in your family became sick, who would care for him or her? Are the caretakers males or females? Why?

2. Think about how you cope with day-to-day events. Is this different to coping with more substantial demands? If so, in what ways? Why do you think this is?

3. Recall a situation where you did not feel in control and felt threatened. How did you react? Did you do anything to alter the situation?

4. How much do you depend on the support of others in difficult times? Write down a list of people who are (a) the most frequent providers of support for you, (b) provide the most substantial support in times of need, and (c) the nature of the support they provide. Are these people the same, or do different people meet different support needs? Why do you think this is?

5. Draw a small circle at the centre of a page, representing your-self. Now, think about a problem in your personal life. Draw radial lines from the circle representing yourself to other circles rep-resenting people who provide you with support. Make the lines connecting those people shorter; the more support they provide, the closer their circle should be to yours. Try to organize these people into social units; family, friends, work colleagues, etc.

6. Repeat the exercise described in 4, but this time select a work-related problem. How is the pattern different?

4

Components of Communication

By the end of this chapter, you should be able to:

- list the main components of communication

- describe the contribution of these components to effective communication

- recognize the importance of context in communications

- recognize what is meant by jargon and its influence in communication

- explain what is meant by a language community

- describe the nature and role of belief systems

- describe the concept of world view

Introduction

Conventionally, we distinguish two main aspects of face-to-face communication: vocalizations (speech and non-speech sounds called para-linguistic utterances); and non-verbal behaviour ('body language' and everything else). Vocalizations and body language are synchronized: when one person is speaking the other person generally is silent, their behaviour is synchronous with the conversation.

In Chapter 2 we concluded that many factors influence the final meaning derived by a listener, not simply the words spoken. Expectations and past experience of the listener, the relationship of the listener to the speaker, the current concerns of the listener, among other things, influence the meaning experienced by the listener. Physical, social and psychological contexts exert profound influence upon the meaning of a message. Indeed, context makes meaningful communication possible. Considerable assumptions are made about the nature of the message, particularly its verbal content, as the rate of information flow during speech is too great for each word to be recognized from scratch; there are simply too many possibilities at any moment. The rules of grammar help considerably by restricting the possible development of a sentence structure within manageable limits. Many of these issues are considered more closely in the present chapter.

Components of communication

Verbal components of communication

> 'When I use a word' Humpty Dumpty
> said in a rather scornful tone,
> it means just what I choose it to mean
> — neither more or less.
>
> Lewis Carroll, *Alice in Wonderland*

Humpty Dumpty's insistence is very reasonable. The use of speech relies on long and extensive learning in childhood. Speech begins to appear very early (Richards, 1974). By six months of age, a child produces predominantly the phonemes (speech sounds) characteristic of the language(s) spoken in its environment (Birdwhistell, 1972).

A child learns that things are to be considered as separate from one another rather than as an interpenetrating whole, and then that these separate things all have names. This view is encouraged by the nature of the grammar underlying Western, particularly English, languages (Bohm,

1980). Grammar adds meaning as this example of verse from *The Jabberwock* by Lewis Carrol illustrates:

> 'Twas brilig, and the slivey toves
> Did gyre and gimble in the wabe,
> All mimsy were the borogoves,
> And the mome raths outgabe.

Though often considered nonsense verse, *The Jabberwock* demonstrates how constrained we are in being able to make words mean different things. Though novel creations, 'slithey toves', 'wabe', 'borogoves' and 'mome raths' have the character of nouns by their location. Similarly, 'gyre','gimble' and 'outgabe' all have the flavour of verbs. So where Humpty Dumpty was in some sense correct, he is, like the rest of us, restricted by the grammar structuring language.

In addition to the formal words and grammar of a given language, other speech sounds, not strictly linguistic elements, add or modify meaning. Pauses, emphasis of breathing, 'uhm's, 'ah's and 'er's, tonal nuances and intonation or expression form what are known as para-linguistic utterances. These non-word sounds punctuate our speech and enrich meaning. A cough at a certain point in a conversation can signal caution, incredulity or surprise. A sigh similarly communicates fatigue, impatience, or even desperation. Pronounced 'er's in a conversation may signal uncertainty or unwillingness, while 'huh' can imply distain in English.

While people in a community may all speak a common language, they will not all share the same understanding or meaning. Meaning can be called trans-linguistic as a result.

During conversation both parties often assume to know what is being discussed when they actually have different interpretations. Blumhagen (1984) gives the example of hypertension meaning high blood pressure to health workers, but to some American people it implies raised muscle tension. Both doctors and patients 'understood' the word but it had very different meaning to each. Misunderstandings like this are particularly problematic in health care settings where patients may be totally unfamiliar with the most basic knowledge and procedures. Nurses or doctors, by contrast, are very familiar with health care and tend to assume incorrectly that everyone else is too.

Ambiguity of meaning can be used to good effect. For example when assessing a patient, a nurse may say, 'Are you finding it difficult?' without clarifying what difficulty is referred to, leaving patients to raise any feature of their circumstances they may be having problems with.

Jargon, specialist languages and language communities

Language itself is more than a set of utterances. Most people raised in China speak Putonghua. Yet, within each community, different variants of Putonghua are used (though many of these are now disappearing due to urbanization, population mobility and mass media). Language variants are called dialects. Dialects give identity to social and cultural subgroups within each community. A dialect indicates if a person is local or otherwise. Unfamiliarity with some dialects excludes strangers from the community. Communities are not just defined geographically. They are found in all segments of society. Many occupational subgroups have their own language which communicates specialist knowledge as well as signalling membership.

These are called language communities. Examples of language communities are seen in the use of medical language — 'medicalese' — among health care workers, the use of legal jargon — 'legalese' — among the legal fraternity, 'militarese' used by members of the armed forces, 'street jive' — the variant of English spoken by poor urban North American Blacks, 'BBC English', Cockney rhyming slang, and so on. A person's speech style is both a means to communicate with others and a badge of membership to a particular group within society. These groups in turn are seen to possess status characteristics, and so language also signals social status.

Most patients are unfamiliar with the most basic aspects of hospitals. They are also in a foreign community, unfamiliar with the language used. Health workers speak medical jargon. 'Jargon' refers to words, terms and neologisms used in the limited domain of (in this case) health care, but rarely used outside it. Examples are many; 'primigravida', 'hypoglycemic', in fact almost all medical, and most nursing, terms are not well understood by patients, deriving as many do from Latin or Greek.

Many terms are widely used by both health workers and patients: 'depression', 'hypertension', 'D and C', but they may not have the same meaning in the lay and medical mind. Specialist languages have evolved to enable effective and precise communication of often highly technical material between fellow workers in a given occupational group. Part of medical and nursing education is to learn the language of health care, medicalese. Technical terms are often necessary for precision in health care. Most patients don't speak or understand medicalese and many health workers overlook this, which is a problem!

Patients are excluded from equality in health care exchanges by many factors including jargon. They are excluded even further in some health care settings, especially where English (the international language of medicine) is not the native language of the patients. Doctors on ward rounds in Hong Kong often insist on discussing the patient's condition with colleagues in English to exclude the patient.

Non-verbal components of communication

> Don't look at me, Sir,
> with - ah - in that tone of voice.
>
> *Punch* (1884)

Non-verbal communication has been closely studied with elaborate choreographic techniques, similar to those used to script dance movement. These record precisely the movement that occurs when individuals attempt to communicate. *Intention* to communicate is not necessary; the presence of another person is enough to affect our behaviour. We may look at them, or ignore them, subtly or obviously. In so doing we communicate information about ourselves. Waiting rooms are good places to observe low-level interchanges such as brief eye-contact and slight smiles, or no smiles and hard looks. Information on body posture has been popularized, particularly for 'reading' other peoples' thoughts and feelings, and how to begin relationships at parties, and in management or business.

Non-verbal behaviour represents the foundation of communication. It is difficult to falsify non-verbal behaviour well, unlike verbal communication when anything can be said, whether it be true or not. Hence the saying, 'actions speak louder than words'. Indeed we honour those skilled in non-verbal roles as actresses and actors. So it is in health care. Anxious patients display characteristic behaviours, such as restlessness, scanning of the environment, or tense expressions. The nurse who doesn't make eye-contact with a patient communicates lower accessibility to one who does. A doctor who doesn't look at a patient during an abdominal examination communicates something different than the doctor who does, and so on.

To illustrate this, list three non-verbal behaviours which:
1. put you off talking with a stranger
2. encourage you to talk to a stranger

Appearance

First impressions are important in communications. Stereotypes influence first impressions and we categorize people throughout our day-to-day lives in terms of such impressions. Dress and grooming communicates a great deal about ourselves. Our appearence communicates our age, gender, sometimes our roles, value systems, our wealth and social status. These influence subsequent conversations, providing cues for dominance in conversation and related social heirarchy in the interaction process.

Thus, a conversation between two people of approximately equal age and dress may proceed in a slightly competetive manner in order to establish dominance within the conversation. Alternatively, there may be a shying away from conversation, or talking about neutral subjects, attempting to find common interests, such as sport. Dress one of these people in a designer suit, gold watch and expensive shoes, dress the other in ragged clothes and the down-dressed person is likely to experience difficulty in achieving equality in the conversation. This applies to both men and women.

Differences in appearance are reduced by wearing uniforms, which is one reason why schools, military and health care establishements insist on uniforms. A person in a health care setting wearing a white coat, open or closed, and displaying a stethoscope is almost certainly a doctor. If the white coat is crumpled and the pockets stuffed with papers, notebooks, pens and patella hammers, then the doctor is almost certainly a junior doctor. If the white coat is crisp and well pressed, and the pockets almost empty, a more senior doctor is indicated. If a business suit is worn, while accompanied by either a nurse or doctor in a white coat, then the person is almost certainly a consultant, or a non-medical official.

Nurses wear military-style rank indicators, such as different stripes on the cap, epaulets or different coloured uniform. Uniforms both protect nurses and doctors from blood and infectious agents and also indicate role and status. The latter is more effectively achieved than the former. This information helps us decide what level of interaction is appropriate.

Eye-contact

Two elements of non-verbal behaviour are very important. These are eye-contact and touch. Eye-contact is probably the most powerful non-verbal behaviour for initiating, maintaining and breaking-off communication.

Eye-contact occurs when two peoples' gaze meet. It is a very primitive and important communication behaviour. A person who stares indicates variously aggression, dominance, intense interest, uncertainty, sadness or affection. Minute variation in the type and context of the gaze differentiates these different meanings. With eye-contact communication occurs from facial and contextual cues. Eye-contact may increase a sense of tension or arousal quite spontaneously and quickly.

Consider the following conversational exchange during a clinical visit to the patient's bedside. (In this and all subsequent examples, HW indicates the health worker, while Pt.(/Rel.) indicates the patient (relative)).

Health worker walks to foot of patient's bed, picks up patient's chart and begins to study it.

HW: How are you today?
Pt: Not bad.
HW: Any pain?

Pt: No.

HW: (Looking at patient for the first time during conversation) Good. Look's like all's well.

Pt: Hmm.

HW: I'll drop by to see you tomorrow. Bye.

Pt: Bye.

Is this a satisfactory exchange? If so, how do you know this? If not, how do you know? Some would feel this was not satisfactory, the patient communicating this by his terse comment. One reason is that the doctor does not make eye-contact until the interview is almost over. He is busy with other things (the patient's chart), and the patient, correctly, objects to this.

Conversational eye-contact in an allopathic health care setting may have the following pattern: speaker makes and breaks eye-contact at will but generally gazes at the mouth, eyes, hands of the listener. They may look extensively at the surroundings while speaking. The listener watches the eyes, mouth and to a lesser extent the hands of the speaker almost exclusively. The listener looking away from the speaker immediately indicates loss of attention, interest or other rejection of communication. Thus, a physician who reads case notes while the patient talks will automatically indicate disinterest in the patient and the patient will reduce, if not cease, talking almost at once.

Touch

Touch is physical contact between two people. Every person is sensitive to a personal space around his or her body. Personal space varies from a few centimeters to two or more feet out from the surface of the body. Personal space varies according to culture, gender, age, roles of a person and nature of interaction, and the characteristics of the person being interacted with. When personal space is encroached, a person may feel very differently depending on the circumstances of the encroachment. Personal space also includes the psychological spaces of familiarity and privacy.

Where the other person enters one's personal space it is called intimacy. Intimacy is very appropriate and important in normal human relationships between close individuals. However, where intimacy is from a stranger or non-related person, say on a crowded bus or train, alternative avoidant behaviours occur. Women place arms across the front of the body, covering the breasts or holding a bag over the pelvic region, and avoid eye-contact. It is very difficult to make eye-contact for more than a brief period with a person in a crowded commuter train, for example because the encroachment of body space. Certain parts of the body, principally those with sexual associations require a wider clearance than other parts.

Touch can communicate care and concern, affection, pain or aggression. In health care, two types of touch are primarily used: touch associated with diagnosis or treatment, such as palpation of the abdomen, and touch that might be used to offer concern, reassurance, support or empathy.

Both types of touch use eye-contact and context to differentiate meaning. In a physical examination, a physician usually looks either at the part of the body being palpated or examined, or elsewhere, if the patient is of the opposite sex. This is more likely if the part of the body being examined has sexual associations. Prolonged eye-contact together with touch often will imply sexual interest. In order to remove any suggestion of sexual contact, the physician or nurse will avoid making eye-contact with the patient, except to very briefly check the patient's facial expression for indications of pain or discomfort perhaps. Males tend to touch females more than the other way round, but there are no gender differences in the touching of children by adults (Major, Schmidlin and Williams, 1990).

During a physical examination, deliberate avoidance of eye-contact indicates respect and non-intimacy. Consider the same exchange, this time between a doctor and a patient of the opposite sex about a surgical wound in the groin. Doctor pulls down sheets and opens the patient's clothes,

HW: How are you today?
Pt: Not bad.
HW: Any pain?
Pt: No.
HW: (Looking at patient for the first time during conversation) Good. Look's like all's well.
Pt: Hmm.
HW: I'll drop by to see you tomorrow. Bye.
Pt: Bye.

This exchange is slightly more acceptable given the changed context. But the doctor correctly avoids eye-contact to avoid the emotion normally associated with the intimacy of one person touching the belly of another of the opposite sex.

Touch indicating care, concern, support or empathy very powerfully supplements emotionally ladened aspects of health communications. Unfortunately, these communications are infrequent.

One reason is that health workers and patients are often not physically close when they talk, which makes reaching out a hand difficult. Touching is also determined by gender and cultural rules. Health workers and patients from different cultural backgrounds touch much less because of uncertainty over its appropriateness, or fear of misinterpreted intent. Patients may see this as discrimination, a cold, uncaring manner, or precisely the opposite!

Cultural or religious prohibitions to touch tend to stop health workers touching patients all together for non-diagnostic or treatment reasons, rather than limiting their touch to appropriate situations.

Touching for concern or support may involve holding hands or touching an arm or a shoulder. This may be prolonged or brief in duration. This can communicate powerfully your concern or empathy with the patient. Sometimes, when there seems little to say, such as with a recently bereaved relative, touch like this can be the most appropriate form of communication.

During this kind of touch, eye-contact is much more common and though not prolonged, occurs from time to time.

Posture and gesture

Posture is the way we hold our bodies, and gestures are what we do with our bodies and limbs to punctuate or accentuate certain things we say. Gesture is much more intentional in terms of desire to communicate than is posture, in most cases.

Body posture indicates openness (arms and legs uncrossed), defensiveness (arms/legs crossed, legs crossed against other person), relaxation (leaning back), interest (leaning forward), and other moods and attitudes. Conversation between people feeling at ease with each other show mirroring of their postures. Both bodies may lean in the same direction, or a hand may support the head, etc. This is called postural echo; it signals agreement and sharing non-verbally. Postural echo is effective in helping to put another person at ease. It is a powerful technique for building rapport.

Gesture serves to complement verbal exchanges, but many gestures have their own meanings. These vary from culture to culture, though some are becoming universal. Examples are the thumbs up gesture for affirmation, or lifting the shoulders with the palms of the hands turned up (shrug) — I don't know; too bad. Gestures help to turn a dry verbal exchange into an animated and richly expressive conversation.

Context

Non-verbal components of communication are learned during initiation into the social world during our early childhood. Later, we learn meanings may change with context. For example, a joke which causes laughter in one social circumstance may be frowned upon in another as inappropriate, flippant or childish. Thus, a nurse jokes with a patient to help relieve anxiety prior to an operation, but post-operatively joking may not be appreciated, and might receive a very different response.

As an illustration of how context changes the meaning of a particular message, consider the following two exchanges between nurse and patient:

Setting: patient recovering from uneventful elective surgery.
Example 1.

Nurse: Can I take your blood pressure please? (Making eye-contact)
Pt: (Extending arm) If I've got any left. (Laughing)
N: Let's see, shall we? (Applying cuff and taking reading)
N: Yes, you've still got a drop or two left. (Smiling)
Pt: They've take so much out of me these last two days, I'm surprised!
N: (Trying to write BP on chart) Oh look, I've broken the clip!

Now, consider the following exchange.
Example 2.

N: Can I take your blood pressure please?'(Looking at sphygmomanometer)
Pt: (Extending arm, smiling)
N: (Applying cuff and taking reading)
Pt: Have I got any left? (Looking at nurse)
N: (Trying to write BP on chart) Oh look, I've broken the clip!.

In these two exchanges, the context and therefore the meaning of the last phrase is different. Can you say how? Would the two conversations now develop differently? Which will be more beneficial?

The meaning transmitted to the patient from the final statement of the nurse will differ considerably. In Example 1, the statement on 'the clip' is part of an ongoing exchange, and is thus not inappropriate, the nurse having established a good rapport and conversational style with the patient. So in Example 1, the nurse invites the patient to share her 'broken clip problem'. Example 2 begins differently with the nurse maintaining distance by not making eye-contact, and generally responding in a more business-like manner all round. This nurse fails to establish rapport with the patient, no conversation occurs and the statement about the clip is made to herself. She is interested in a task but not the patient. The patient is a passive recipient of a procedure.

The context in this example is not a place, but a style of relationship. Generally, health care or hospital contexts make patients feel disadvantaged and somewhat threatened. Patients may be unfamiliar with basic issues, they do not belong to the hospital 'community', they do not understand the many lines of communication or hierarchies that exist. Things overheard or misunderstood may be interpreted in the worst possible way by patients made anxious by the hospital/illness context.

Belief systems and conflicting interpretations

World views

Personal beliefs and expectations about how life, the universe and everything fit together, and the nature of the interactions between ourselves and the world are held by everyone. A world view is the personally perceived causal context of someone's existence. Each person's 'world view' develops from his or her own unique set of experiences and so is different from the next person's world view. World views of people raised within the same culture, subculture and social group are often different. The world views of people raised in different cultures can be drastically different.

Social groups are largely responsible for instilling the value systems of particular cultures. These value systems are the sum of many generations of a particular social group's values and beliefs. We adopt a world view by using this cultural value system to interpret what happens to us.

If, for example, the value system of a community maintained that after death the spirits of the departed remained present but invisible, then spirit possession may be believed possible. Then it offers one credible explanation for certain behaviour. Alternatively, value systems emphazising biological/material values demand an explanation for forms of unacceptable behaviour to be made in disease terms. Spirit possession is thus dismissed as 'superstition'.

Many cultural value systems offer rich explanations of how the universe works. These systems include subcultural systems such as medicine (Spicker and Ratzan, 1990). Two very different such value systems are the Western scientific world view and the traditional Chinese world view. In terms of understanding and explaining illness within a culture, the predominant Western view is reductionist and mechanistic. The body is seen as a complex machine, and disease as breakdown or malfunction of this machine. Thus, molecular spanners and micro-adjustments of sub-systems are obvious tools to use to fix the malfunctioning machine. The mechanical parallel is clear.

In contrast, the traditional Chinese world view is one example of holistic world views. A person requires constant balance and flow of energy (Ch'i) in and out and through set pathways within the body, like an electric circuit. If this energy flow is reduced or excessive in places, or where the overall level of energy is deficient, specific manifestations of symptoms and ill-health appear. Treatment balances energy, its level and flow. Manipulating energy nodes can enhance or redirect the flow. Moreover, food has both energy giving and removing qualities, so a balanced diet is required to maintain a balance of health, and so on.

These simplified descriptions illustrate how different world views of illness causality may be. A patient with traditional Chinese views of illness may first make a dietary change, or seek herbal medicines. This may be followed by perhaps acupressure, acupuncture or moxibustion. The patient may perceive certain types of Western treatment (such as injections) as more potent than others (such as tablets), and will agree to the use of the former as a last resort or when a speedy 'cure' is required (Lo et al, 1994).

These examples illustrate very extensive differences in world view, but less obvious ones can be found within a culture. Doctors or nursees who fail to consider the patient's world view is assuming they and their patient hold the same view of ill health. Seldom will this be the case. Such differences in world views may influence the extent treatment will be accepted or complied with (Fielding, 1987).

In other cases, the patient's world view may contain powerful implications about certain illnesses. Cancer is seen as implying certain death within Italian culture (Gordon, 1990). In the United States, cancer has been described as holding a status similar to that of tuberculosis in nineteenth-century Europe, one related to repression of the passions (Sontag, 1977).

Summary

Face-to-face communication is highly complex. Verbal messages, punctuated with para-linguistic utterances may be reinforced, or contradicted by non-verbal behaviours. Specialist language developed to deal with the technical aspects of contemporary health care has also created a health care fraternity which excludes patients. Use of jargon deceives health workers, who fail to consider that patients are excluded, both in terms of knowledge and also social participation. When you are lying down, it is difficult to talk with someone looking down on you and using words you do not understand.

In attempts to involve the patient as an equal participant, health workers often fail to consider the patient's differing world view.

In summary, many problems in health care communications derive from basic differences between backgrounds of the participants. This fundamental point is often overlooked, but is extremely important. Health workers must attempt to minimize differences in communication arising from differences in background. Otherwise, all the more subtle skills will be to no avail.

Exercises

1. Observe how people present themselves physically at work. Look for posture, gesture and personal space. Try and identify open and closed postures which indicate accessibility and protection. How do gestures change when accompanied with such postures?

2. Observe the way that people behave during different types of conversation. When one speaks how does the other behave? Do they take turns or do they speak in some other form of dialogue? How do different situations, relationships and activities affect spoken exchanges, if at all?

3. During your work, observe how colleagues interact with their patients. Who speaks when? What might influence these patterns? How do colleagues' moods affect their behaviour?

4. Find a partner with whom you can do some simple exercises. One of you speaks, while the other looks elsewhere, not paying attention. Try this for a few moments, change roles, then discuss how you feel. Why do you think you felt the way you did?

5. Try touching your partner's face while talking about your favourite activity. Do the same thing while asking about some personal aspect of your partner's life. Are there differences in how it feels to talk under these circumstances? How does your partner feel? Discuss what might influence these feelings.

5

Starting the Interview

Educational Objectives

By the end of this chapter, you should be able to

- identify the three stages of a clinical interview
- explain what is meant by manifest or overt and latent or covert goals of consultation
- recognize examples of the six different question forms used by health workers
- identify the question styles used by health workers that are most desirable from the patient's perspective
- recognize the interview stage during which patients are most likely to ask questions
- recognize the interview stage where patients are most likely to be passive
- list the communication components involved in beginning an interview
- recognize the effects of business-like and friendly behaviour by the doctor on the patient's level of satisfaction with the consultation
- recognize the advantages and disadvantages in explaining the time available for interview

Introduction

The term 'clinical interview' refers to health worker-patient interactions. This may be a formal interview, such as a patient consultation, or admission interview. Much of the research carried out on clinical interviews has focused on out-patient interviews rather than in-patient interviews. Here a mixture of examples will be used.

Models of consultation

Friedson (1961, 1970a,b) developed a model of consultation on the principle of general conflict negotiation. Friedson (1970b) believed this model to apply to all relationships between all types of clinical professionals and their patients. The model rests on the assumption that the interaction between patient and health worker is based on conflict, which is inherent because patients and health workers both have different perspectives. This difference in perspective may be aggrevated by important differences in manifest goals (presenting problem) and latent goals (real problem) of the patient and health worker (Ben Zira, 1980). As a result of the conflict, Friedson (1970a) proposed that patient-health worker interaction necessarily involves negotiation of separate conditions, perspectives and understandings. That is, both health worker and patient may have different goals they wish to achieve, and just as in industrial conflicts over pay and conditions, negotiation is required to establish mutually agreeable goals, and to define and manage the patient's problem (see Chapter 7).

So interview participants have different goals. During a regular visit to an out-patient clinic for diabetes check-up, staff need to check the patient's glucose control and screen for vascular complications. The patient seeks feedback and advice on problem management and ways to minimize adverse consequences of the disease (Bryant, McFarland and Michels, 1990). Thus, the consultation must reconcile these differing needs if both parties are to be satisfied.

For example, interviewing a patient admitted with chest pain to a Coronary Care Unit lays the basis for a care plan. But the patient seeks information, reassurance, control of anxiety and pain and the development of trust. Physiotherapy assessment involves gathering data on patients' abilities and problems, but the patient may want information on type and expected duration of treatment and effects on lifestyle. Finally, patients hospitalized for surgery benefit from being interviewed both by a surgeon and anaesthetist. One recent study found that while more than a third of patients had fears about the anaesthetic, a third did not receive a visit from the surgeon beforehand (van Wijk and Smalhout, 1990).

Structure of the interview

The clinical interview has three phases: the taking of a history; a physical or similar examination; and a discussion of findings and proposed treatment.

The history

The goal of the medical history for the health worker is to establish a diagnosis of a patient's problems (Cicourel, 1975; 1978; 1980). This tends to be achieved most readily in relation to the patient's manifest goal (the presenting problem), but there may be a failure to achieve resolution of the patient's latent goal (the motivation for the consultation) (Ben Zira, 1980). Chapter 1 discussed the failure of many clinical interviews to detect underlying psychological or emotional elements, related or unrelated to the patient's presenting problem. Resolution of these is often the patient's latent goal. These are particularly likely to be overlooked when the patient presents with an identifiable physical disorder.

Not identifying the patient's main problems leads to an incomplete database upon which clinical decisions about the problem and treatment are made. Diagnostic errors which thus arise are at best a waste of resources and at worst a potential hazard to the patient.

In order to identify problems, a health worker uses various reasoning processes. The physician's database consists of medical intelligence and clinical experience. These must be applied to the identification of a set of specific and effective questions, the answers to which will distinguish between competing hypotheses about the patient's diagnosis. Simultaneously, health workers must integrate the patient's specific experiential information with that of their own technical database. A study by Hampton et al (1975) indicated that this is a highly effective means of deriving diagnoses, when done appropriately. In 82% of cases studied, diagnoses were made on the basis of the history alone, while the physical examination and other investigations lead to a diagnosis in only 9% each of the remaining cases studied. If the database is incomplete, however, accurate diagnosis is much less likely, causing a failure of the consultation process and an unsatisfactory interview all round.

The practitioner often does not know in advance what is wrong with the patient. Nonetheless, hypothesis formation about problems begins very early in the interview. As the perceptual system seeks confirmatory evidence and is less sensitive to contradictory evidence, practitioners try to confirm their hypothesis (Ng, 1991), rather than to refute it (Lanes, 1988). The information to test these hypotheses is elicited by a question-answer sequence. Sinclair and Coulthard (1975) defined six different question forms used by health workers:

1. Yes-No interrogative questions; e.g. 'Got any pain?'
2. Questions with answers/ interrogative questions; e.g. 'Did they say what it was? Was it your tummy?'
3. Forced-choice interrogatives; e.g. 'How did it feel? Was it sharp, dull, throbbing?'
4. Tag-Questions, two-part interrogatives; e.g. 'The pain was the same as the first time, was it?'
5. Requests for confirmation declaratives; e.g. 'So the pain comes on *after* your meals?'
6. Requests for more information on certain topics; e.g. 'Tell me about the pain now.'

The first five questions pressure the patient to respond in the way that the health worker wants, or needs, in order to make sense of the personal experience of the patient. If the patient fully conforms to responding in the manner expected of him, then the negotiation is conducted in the perspective of the health worker. The risk here is that the patient may tell the practitioner what he or she wants to hear, which may not be accurate. There is considerable social pressure on patients to be seen to be 'good' patients. 'Good' translates as cooperative rather than accurate.

Only when a request for information is made to the patient (question form 6) is the patient encouraged to express information from a personal perspective. Drass (1982) reported only 29% of questions asked in the history-taking phase of clinical interviews were were non-restrictive requests for information: 71% of questions were restrictive in nature. However, in 40% of cases, responses to these restrictive questions were expansions or indirect replies, suggesting patients were not happy at the one-sided perspective the interview was taking.

Restrictive questioning enables health workers to introduce discriminative questions to the patient, which, together with the answers, provide a structural framework for applying the database of general medical knowledge to an individual case (Drass, 1982). By contrast, patients seem to resist these attempts to 'generalize' their illness experiences by adding further information which they believe is important. Patients also correct health workers when the latter's general assumptions are perceived as inappropriate.

The examination

The second phase of the interview is the physical examination phase. Not all clinical interviews require a physical examination. When used, the physical examination serves to elicit physical signs. These may serve a number of purposes. For example, as clues to the patient's medical problem, or to confirm the status of a nursing site, such as pressure sore or surgical wound. This would occur, for example, prior to planning care, or to assess the functional capacity of a limb before implementing a physiotherapy programme. Hence, in this context physical signs serve as directly perceived signs of health status.

The physical examination has two notable communications features. First, the examination is largely a non-verbal data gathering exercise. Second, verbal communications tend to be dominated by the health worker, with more than three times as many verbal acts as are seen from the patient (Drass, 1982). These verbal communications tend to be in the form of statements from health worker to patient requesting non-verbal acts. Directives constitute 48% of these (Drass, 1982), such as 'breathe deeply', 'turn to a lateral position', or 'walk'. Verbal acts from the patient tend almost always (93%, Drass, 1982) to be responses to questions from the health worker. It follows that for the physical examination to be useful, the patient must cooperate.

The physical examination is notable for the degree of body contact. In the context of the physical examination, such contact is referred to as diagnostic touching (Pratt and Mason, 1984), though other kinds of touching may occur (incidental or accidental touching, for example). Touching is almost usually seen as appropriate by patients. This is so even if the most socially sensitive interactions, such as vaginal examination by a male doctor, are involved. Physical examinations are perceived as highly important by health workers, especially physiotherapists (Pratt and Mason, 1984). This serves as another excellent illustration of context on the meaning of communication (Chapter 4).

The problem discussion

The third phase of the clinical interview is the problem-discussion phase. A medical, nursing or other diagnosis means the health worker has conceptualized the patient's problem in terms of the health worker's professional expertise. During this phase of the interview, 64% of the verbal acts from the health worker provide information to the patient. Patients are seldom asked to respond to these instructions verbally. Health workers rely more on non-verbal cues and look for acknowledgment of the information.

Patients may interject questions of their own at any stage of the interview, but during the discussion phase, patient-selected questions account for about 45% of patient verbal acts, more frequently than during examination (11% of patient verbal acts), or history taking phases (0.6% of patient verbal acts) (Drass, 1982).

During the history-taking phase, patients raise their own questions or provide information when questioned by the health worker in a turn-taking pattern. However, during the physical examination, either party may be doing things that make speech difficult, e.g. holding breath, listening through a stethoscope, or be out of line of sight of the patient. Also, the patient is often in the horizontal position; this is a particularly socially submissive position for challenging communication dominance with a health worker standing over the patient. Also, as the health worker is utilizing professional expertise this is not seen as an appropriate time for the patients to voice their opinion (Drass, 1982). After all, it is this expertise the patient has come to consult.

Patient-selected questions are often attempts at individualizing what might otherwise be a general discussion. This is particularly true in the discussion phase, where the health worker may present the patient's problem as an example of a general category of problems. Patients may prefer discussion to be more about their unique problem and treatment as a individualized event. Patients frequently complain that health workers are more interested in the patients' problems than in the patients themselves. Attempts by patients to individualize the discussion of their problem may reflect patients' desires to make themselves the object of the discussion rather than their problem.

Drass (1982) argued that the context of the discussion in clinical interviews changes according to the stage of the interview. The movement from one stage of interview to another is controlled by the health worker who has an explicit need to progress from history-examination-discussion in order to fully utilize professional expertise. The patient, on the other hand, already possesses information on the condition, though of a personal kind. It seems then, from what we know of patient responses to illness and of research like that described by Drass (1982), that the patient may be more interested in understanding or making sense out of the illness during the discussion phase of the interview.

If the patient asks for information or volunteers information relating to his or her concerns, the patient is speaking out of context. These out of context questions and comments are responded to in one of three ways by the health workers. They may stop and address the patient's question. They may choose to ignore, or interrupt the comment, or indicate that discussion of that point is inappropriate at the time it was raised by the patient. Health workers tend to use the ignoring or interrupting response most (Drass, 1982).

This is important, for if patients are to have any impact upon diagnostic decisions, they must know not only what to say (that is, have a legitimate medical explanation), but when to say it (Drass, 1982).

Interview style

Buller and Buller (1987) have identified two general styles used in clinical interviews that they have called affiliation and control.

Behaviours characterizing the affiliative style include those which communicate interest, friendliness, empathy, warmth, genuineness, candour, honesty, compassion, a desire to help, devotion, sympathy, authenticity, an non-judgmental attitude, humour and a social orientation (Buller and Buller, 1987). By contrast, behaviours characterizing the controlling style of interaction communicate power, control, authority, professional detachment and status (Friedson, 1970; Ben Zira, 1980).

Interaction style strongly affects patients' evaluation of the effectiveness of health care (Buller and Buller, 1987). Affiliative styles of communication are associated with a more positive evaluation of health care than controlling communication styles in the consultation. The care given by physicians described as dominant/active (those who used more controlling behaviours) is evaluated as poorer than that of less dominant/active practitioners.

However, for patients who perceive themselves as *severely* ill the practitioner's communication style is not associated with evaluation of medical care (Buller and Buller, 1987).

This relationship is unaffected by the patient's age or gender, but younger practitioners seem more likely to be evaluated on the basis of their communication style. Older practitioners are not so readily evaluated by the mostly younger patients (Buller and Buller, 1987).

Techniques for interviewing

Starting the interview

This section outlines some principal points of interviewing styles and techniques. Not all of these approaches will feel right for every student. A standard format has been adopted to describe health worker-patient interactions but individual communication style and interview circumstances may dictate different approaches to those outlined. Use a style that is you. Remember, they are meant to serve as guidelines for practice, not absolute rules that must be strictly adhered to.

A good start to the interview involves the following:
1. introducing self and greeting the client
2. good attitude and friendly manner
3. explanation of purpose of interview/ time available

The consultation can be personalized more by some preliminary exchange between the practitioner and patient before beginning the consultation proper. Willingness to discuss other aspects of a patients' problems can also help to personalize the consultation (Martin and Bass, 1989).

Introducing yourself

On first meeting a person you (or someone else) usually introduce yourself. Many practitioners fail to carry out this most simple task. They incorrectly assume either that the patient already knows who they are or can read their name badges. More extreme opinion is that it is unnecessary or a waste of time. All these assumptions are incorrect. Many hospitals now have 'named nurse' policies, where individualization of caregivers is expected to improve staff-patient relations and patient satisfaction with care given.

At the first meeting, make it standard practice to introduce yourself by name and occupation.

If the interview is taking place in a room, such as a surgery:
- look at the patient as he or she enters
- make eye-contact with the patient
- smile, if appropriate
- make a clear gesture to indicate where the patient is to sit
- as you introduce yourself, make eye-contact
- give your name and title
- give an indication of who you are

e.g.   Hello, I'm Nurse Jane Young. I'm a Health Visitor and I'll be coming to visit you at home after your discharge.

or

Good morning, my name is Edward Low, I'm the doctor who will be looking after you.

or

Please sit down. I am Mary Tam, I'm a radiographer and I would like to talk about the X-ray you'll be having.

For young children and elderly patients, it may be necessary to introduce yourself in an age-appropriate manner at the first few meetings. With teenage, adult and aware elderly patients, this should not be necessary.

Always address young children directly if they are the patient.

If you are seeing the patient for the first time, avoid looking at the case notes or other records where possible while the patient is in the room. It is especially important,

NOT to gesture to the patient without making eye-contact

NOT to keep the patient waiting in silence while reading the patient's notes, especially on entry

NOT to use a patronizing manner with patients

NOT to assume the patient knows who you are, what the interview is for, or how long it will last

Consultations initiated by the patient obviously contradict to some extent the last point. It may be that the health worker does not know what the patient's problem is, as in the case of a patient-initiated consultation in a primary care facility.

Avoid seating arrangements with the following characteristics:

- where you sit behind a desk
- where you are higher/lower than the patient
- where you are too close or too far away from the patient
- where you face the patient directly

Good seating arrangements will be

- at right angles to each other, so it is easy for both to look away if they wish
- on the same level and type of seating as the patient (the same level is especially important for children, people in bed or wheelchairs)
- at a comfortable distance from the patient so quiet speech can be heard
- where you can reach out and touch the patient's hand if necessary

Key Points

Effectively introducing yourself and explaining who you are communicates consideration to the patient. It requires a certain:

- skill
- attitude
- affiliative style

The attitude of the health worker is all important. It is imperative to establish an atmosphere where patients feel they are a participant in the health care process with an approachable health worker (Brody, 1980; Korsch et al,1968; Ley, 1977; Schulman, 1979).

Establishing rapport

Rapport refers to relationship, connection or being in sympathy with another person's communication attempts. It is important to establish rapport before launching into the main body of the interview. Once established, rapport can be built upon as the interview proceeds. (The topic of rapport is dealt with further in Chapter 8.)

A common way to establish rapport is, following the introduction, to ask the client briefly about topics which indicate respect and interest in the patient as a person.

HW: I hope you weren't kept waiting long? We're a bit short of staff, all away on holiday.
Pt: No. It doesn't matter.
HW: Are you on holiday right now?
Pt: No, we went away at Easter this year, to China.
HW: Hope the weather was better for you than it is now.
Pt: Yes, it was.
HW: Well, is there anything I can do for you?

This patient is not very forthcoming. The health worker correctly moves on to the reasons for consultation, but some rapport has been established and this can be built on later.

To establish rapport with children, it is useful to talk about their interests in an enthusiastic way. Common interests can also be acknowledged by the health worker. This is a useful technique to use with adolescents also.

Business-like or friendly?

Are patients more satisfied with a business-like health worker than with a friendly one? Research consistently confirms preference for a friendly manner (Ley, 1977; Thorne, 1993). Building up a good relationship with the patient require *affiliative behaviours*. Of course, friendly people are more approachable than business-like people and more comfortable to be with. Approachability can be enhanced by two lines of strategy.

The first strategy is by being friendly, which is enhanced by:
• introducing yourself by your full name rather than 'Doctor Young' or 'Nurse Lee'; then adding your profession, if needed
• smiling and being interested in the patient
• engaging in some non-medical talk
• treating the patient with respect and concern

The second strategy is by encouraging patients to take some responsibility for the consultation, which may be done by:
* asking what the patient expects from the interview
* encouraging patient involvement in negotiating interview goals
* active listening
* providing adequate information

It is important to improve approachability with children. Children in medical settings are a special and vulnerable group. They are in unfamiliar surroundings. Often, the many psychosocial needs of children are seen as no different to those of adults. Hospitals are seldom user-friendly places for children.

Parents describe a greater sense of professional distance between child patients and hospital staff than with general practitioners (Macaskill and MacDonald, 1982). Medical staff tend to be seen as punitive and non-empathic (Eiser, 1984), and staff empathy may appear dependent on the child's expression of pain for children aged 7 to 10 (Brewster, 1982).

Young children are intimidated by uniforms and white coats. Avoid these when meeting a child for the first time. Uniforms hide individuality and show rank within a moral order. Children have difficulty discriminating between different doctors or nurses. This helps make their perception of their own status ambiguous, increasing existing anxieties.

Have a variety of toys, hand puppets and paper and crayons available to help increase approachability with a young child. If the child has brought along toys into hospital (a good idea), some time might be spent talking about the toy. Sometimes the toy might also be 'sick'. This can be a useful way to bring up the topic of the child's problem.

Key Points

Self-disclosure among children can be facilitated by several consultation factors, including:

* accurate empathy involving the communication of understanding
* non-possessive warmth (the creation of an accepting, safe trusting atmosphere)
* genuineness

Hill (1985) summarized by Wilkinson (1988)

Explanation of the purpose of the interview and time available

Often the patient is not sure about the purpose of an interview, especially during hospitalization. The patient may be visited by many different professionals throughout the day for unknown purposes.

Patients may also be uncertain of the purpose of the interview when referred to a specialist clinic, assessment or treatment centre, or when receiving a home visit. Under these circumstances, some discussion of the purpose of the interview is required.

If the patient presents with a complaint, the interview might aim to gather information on the complaint, to discuss the patient's current concerns or to decide upon a treatment programme.

During an admission interview, a new patient on a hospital ward will expect the admitting nurse to:

- explain the purpose of any procedures and ask permission*
- inquire if the patient understands the purpose of the interview
- suggest that following the procedure, the nurse may answer the patient's questions
- ask if the patient agrees with this format

In a different sort of interview, negotiation of purpose may be needed (see Chapter 7). For example, during an interview with a patient suffering from chronic pain. The health worker may want psychosocial information on the patient while the patient may want relief from pain. To meet both needs, the health worker may suggest that a decision on how to effectively control the pain can only be made with further information. There may then follow discussion of treatment alternatives.

In multi-purpose interviews or when a choice of treatment options exists, it may be helpful for the practitioner to guide or advise the patient.

Where time is short, negotiation is still economical as patient responses are more focused. So, a statement of available time may be made, though some controversy exists regarding this point. Critics claim to do so suggests an unwillingness to spend adequate time with the patient. But it is unrealistic to expect a long consultation where only ten minutes are available.

It is possible to state time available without implying impatience:

HW: We have about ten minutes available. It would be most useful for me if we concentrate first on your legs, then we can decide what the best approach may be. How does that sound?

---

* It should not be necessary to ask if patients understand simple tasks like re-dressing a wound. But the elderly, children and other patients whose understanding may not be good may need a more careful explanation.

Pt: Well, yes.
HW: Is there anything else you wanted to discuss today?
Pt: I did, but . . . (pause)
HW: Would you like to tell me about it?

It is better to avoid placing a time limit on the interview if possible. It is not unusual for patients to raise an important point just as the allocated time is up, leaving the practitioner to extend the interview, or arrange a later interview to discuss the new point.

Summary

Introduction procedure
- look at the patient as he or she enters
- make eye-contact with the patient
- make a clear gesture to indicate where the patient is to sit
- as you introduce yourself, make eye-contact.
- give your name and role
- give an indication of who you are

Facilitating approachability
- introduce yourself using your full name
- smile
- engage in some non-medical talk
- treat the patient with respect and concern
- take an interest in the patient as a person

(and encouraging participation)
- inquire about the patient's goals in the interview
- encouraging patient involvement in negotiating interview goals
- show concern for the impact of the problem on the patient's life
- listen
- providing adequate information

Explanation of purpose and time available
- explain your needs, e.g. data to be gathered
- mention time available
- enquiry if the patient understands the purpose

- suggest that following the procedure, health worker may answer patient's questions
- ask if the patient agrees with this format

or

- inquire what the patient wants to discuss
- explore patient's expectations
- agree upon a common goal for this interview
- suggest an strategy to achieve this

Exercises

Preamble

Two students work together: one takes the role of the health worker and the second the patient. Alternatively, the trainer can produce a teaching tape to illustrate the desired approach before the paired role play. There is no substitute for participation and constructive feedback on performance leads to the most efficient learning. As a minimum, students should role play these exercises in pairs and afterwards spend time discussing how each felt, giving feedback and suggestions for improving performance.

In all these exercises, participants are encouraged to be themselves, responding to the situation as they would respond, except where otherwise directed.

1. *Situation:*   Health worker is in a room/surgery, face to face interview with a new patient. Assume the patient is outside the room. Begin from this point.
    Task: To reach the stage of agreed consultation goal.
    Time available: 5 minutes.
    Health worker: Identify the patient's main problem.
    Patient: Select one of the patient profiles given below.

    Patient profile (a).   You have had repeated headaches for the last week. You have no previous history of headaches. Otherwise your health is good . Work is currently difficult but only mention this if asked.

    Patient profile (b).   You have been having a lot of stomach pains recently which you want sorting out. You drink alcohol almost every night and smoke. Work has meant you don't eat as regularly as you want. Your health has not been good for some time, with tiredness and frequent colds.

Patient profile (c). You think you might be pregnant. (Be yourself, that is single, married etc., where reasonable.)

(Vary this exercise with shorter times.)

2. *Situation:* This patient was admitted today for exploratory abdominal surgery tomorrow.
    Task: To reach agreed interview goal.
    Time available: 5 minute
    Health worker: Do a (brief) admission interview; in this busy surgical unit, there are three other patients awaiting interview and the grand round begins in 15 minutes.
    Patient: Choose one of the patient profiles given.

    Patient profile (a). You have had increasing abdominal pain and discomfort over the last 3 weeks and are anxious about the surgery and pain. You do not know what is involved and want to know.

    Patient profile (b). This is your first hospitalization. You are anxious about why you are here. You were told you needed some tests but not why. Your only symptom is some weight loss.

    Patient profile (c). You have come into hospital for tests. You have been unable to get pregnant for over three years. You hope the doctors will help you.

3. *Situation:* The patient has had some tests, but results are not yet available. The patient is to be discharged today as the bed is needed.
    Task: To agree on interview goals.
    Time available: 5 minutes.
    Health worker: Carry out the discharge interview. Approach the patient in bed or in a side-room.

    Patient profile (a). You have had tests during your three days in hospital but no one has told you the results. You worry that something serious may have been found.

Patient profile (b).   You have spent three days in hospital for tests and want to know if it is all right to return to work.

Patient profile (c).   You are keen to go home after three days in hospital for tests, but are afraid you will get sick again. You want some treatment.

Discussion

These questions serve two goals. First, they stimulate discussion of the above exercises. Consider local cultural or sub-cultural customs that might demand a different approach. Second,they help to identify and resolve attitudinal problems students may have.

1.   Why is it important to involve the patient in the negotiation of interview goals?

2.   Under what circumstances might it be acceptable for the health worker to define the goals without the patient's input?

3.   How friendly versus business-like should the health worker be, when diagnosing a problem and time is short?

4.   To what extent do the practitioner and patient share different goals in the clinical interview?

5.   When time is short, is it acceptable not to negotiate with a patient but to simply go ahead with the questions you want answered?

6

Listening and Questioning

Introduction

This chapter continues the focus on the clinical interview. Here we look more closely at techniques for improving information gathering during clinical interviews. These techniques fall into two groups. First, listening, a basic skill crucial for health workers. Second, the skills of questioning. Specifically, various question forms obtain different types of information. Finally, we look at how to end an interview appropriately.

Listening versus talking

> To hear the message first requires the physician's interest, second his understanding of the meaning of language, and third his sympathy toward and his knowledge and understanding of the circumstances of the patient's life; these again he hears best by listening to the patient.
>
> Pickering (1978)

'Listen to your patient. They will tell you what is wrong with them.' This saying is full of wisdom, but some patients will not tell you directly what is wrong with them. This itself is useful. Unfortunately, health workers spend too little time listening to the patient, and often too much time talking or looking at case notes.

Attending to a speaker is the act we call listening. We cannot listen if we ourselves are talking and, as a rule, others will not talk while we are speaking. Health workers can interfere with the patient giving information by interruption and monologue. The gaze behaviour of physicians significantly influences the amount and type of information patients give. During consultations, when physicians do not look at patients, as when reading case notes, patients cease talking and increase body movement in an attempt to regain the physician's attention. Patients begin talking again when the doctor looks at them once more (Heath, 1984, 1987). The same is likely to occur with a nurse or therapist completing a chart while in conversation with a patient.

Case notes

It is not possible to read and listen to speech concurrently. So if you are reading case notes, you are not listening to the patient. Read case notes before or after an interview. You need to inform the patient that it is necessary. Ask the patient if it is acceptable for you to make notes. If you must have a detailed record of an interview, adapt the session for this. If you need to check notes, say when you are going to do this. Read what you must, then close the notes and resume. Alternatively, allow the patient to explain, then summarize and check for accuracy, then record details.

Listening with your ears

Learning when not to talk is an important communication skill. Listening means attending to what the person is saying. Listening requires occasional questions for guidance. Leave most of the talking to the patient.

In a diagnostic interview a structure and questioning strategy is needed. After negotiating the goals, a good staring point for the interview may be to ask the patient to outline the problem.

> Tell me about why you have come here.
> What do you think I can do to help you?
> What has brought you here today?
> You seem unwell. Would you like to talk about it?

Listen to what is said and not said. The patient may just outline some symptoms. Are they major or minor? If major, how long has the patient had them? If long-standing, why have they mentioned them now? If minor, why is the patient seeking help with them?

Looks for verbal cues in what the patient says and how they say it. Verbal cues exist in:
- emotional content
- pauses
- unwillingness to answer questions
- stuttering
- changes in tone of voice/voice tension

Clarification will be necessary, as when a patient reports feeling depressed or raises anxieties about cancer, for example. Respond in the following manner:

Pt: . . . I was depressed.
HW: What makes you say you were depressed?
or,
Pt: . . . Do you think it might be cancer?
HW: What makes you think of cancer?

Key Points

This questioning format is called *reflective*. It involves reflecting the question back to the patient for elaboration, either by echoing part of the patient's statement:

Pt: . . . so I think it might . . .

(Pause.)

HW: It might . . . ?
Pt: Is it serious? What's wrong with me?

or by a more structured re-presentation of the question to the patient, such as:

Pt: . . . so I think it might . . .

(Pause.)

HW: Might what?
Pt: Is it serious? What's wrong with me?
HW: What makes you think it might be serious?

The tone of voice is very important and should indicate concern. Do not dismiss the patient's concerns.

Listening should illuminate the the patient's perspective. Mentioning cancer may suggest anxiety about the disease. This is informative.

Patients may be very knowledgable about their condition but may be ignored by staff because procedure dictates a different course of action. Remember two things: all patients are different, and patients generally know themselves; in chronic illnesses, patients often know their disease better than most staff.

For example, a diabetic admitted to a coronary care unit (CCU) for angiogram the next day questioned why she needed a 500 mL 5% dextrose drip at 11.00 p.m. She explained to the nurse that she had taken her insulin at 10.00 p.m. and did not normally eat a meal after this, so any further intake of glucose might destabilize her glucose control. The nurse said there was a 'standard procedure' for diabetics having an angiogram.

By morning, the patient was complaining of hyperglycemia. Due to the angiogram, she missed her 8.30 a.m. insulin. On return to the CCU she was given no insulin and a further 500 mL of 5% dextrose solution, despite requesting glucose-free fluid to allow her blood glucose to decline. Again she was told it was 'standard procedure for diabetics'. By late morning the patient was intermittently unconsciousness and distressed. A diabetologist was called to advise on the management of her hyperglycemia. Insulin was given, and her glucose level declined. It took two days of alternate fasting and eating outside meal times to re-schedule her food-insulin intake to breakfast; lunch; dinner. Needless to say, the patient was not pleased.

So, when staff take control from a competent patient, problems may arise. In the example above, failure to listen to the patient precipitated unnecessary disruption of the patient's own health strategies, and caused more risk for the patient, necessitating more nursing and medical care. A clear case of an iatrogenic, or treatment-induced health problem.

By listening and planning treatment with the patient's participation, many problems can be avoided. So can the patients' frustration when their own expertise in themselves is not trusted. Also, in not listening to the patient and removing her control the staff increased the patient's stress.

Children and adolescents

Children and younger adolescents may not say what they feel directly. So *active listening*, hearing expressions of feelings becomes important.

Children often use regressive coping during illness. A previously toilet-trained child may begin to wet the bed at night (*nocturnal enuresis*). Other presenting problems described by parents include children suddenly becoming aggressive or developing abdominal illnesses.

Avoid direct confrontation with the child. Children using regressive coping are doing so because they cannot deal with their demands in more mature ways. Challenging an enuretic child is self-defeating. Instead, look for recent changes in the child's life: school, home, and family (especially changes in parenting practices or in marital harmony) are the three most significant areas. Children may 'act out' traumatic experiences. By utilizing play, it is possible to help clarify any recent events in the child's life. Specialist child services should be consulted if this is required.

Listening with your eyes: non-verbal cues

Non-verbal cues help considerably in consultations. Non-verbal behaviour more than verbal behaviour reflects emotional state. Dysphoria (unhappiness, feeling low, the 'blues') is a common complaint, often presenting as vague physical symptoms. Observing the patient's general behaviour helps in diagnosis of dysphoria. Patients' anxieties about their illness may be indicated by non-verbal cues.

Sometimes you may get a feeling about a patient but are unable to clearly identify what is causing that feeling. It is likely that the patient's non-verbal behaviour is contributing to how you feel.

Non-verbal cues of dysphoria include:
- slow response
- 'sad' countenance
- tearful eyes or tendency to cry easily
- agitation

Some non-verbal indications of worry or anxiety include:
- change in voice, such as increased tremor or stuttering
- increasing restlessness, fidgeting
- nail picking
- tense expression
- increase in pulse in neck
- increased scanning of the environment
- being 'jumpy'
- emphatic swallowing
- appearing 'stuck' when unable to answer questions
- poor attention
- anger or aggressiveness

Embarrassment may be indicated by:
- blushing
- avoiding eye-contact
- appearing 'flustered'
- laughter

Children and adolescents

Young children are often less skilled in hiding feelings by controlling non-verbal behaviour. They usually express feelings, agitation, boredom and other states, being less constrained by social rules.

Adolescents may appear moody but this should not obscure a health worker's sensitivity to acute distress. Many situations trivial to an adult are of significance to adolescents (see Chapter 3). Empathic statements can be used with both children and adolescents to good effect.

> ## Key Points
>
> Sensitivity to both verbal and non-verbal cues is important, especially in medical or nursing diagnosis.
>
> Be aware of what cues you may be transmitting to the patient.
>
> Patients are as skilful as you, in many cases, in 'feeling' your non-verbal response to them.
>
> If you feel disrespectful or angry, most patients will pick this up from your non-verbal behaviour.
>
> *Be accepting*: you are there to provide a service, therefore do not reject your patient.
>
> *Be non-judgemental*: do not pass judgement on your patient. They are not consulting your morals.
>
> *Be warm*: by showing a warm personality, you are more likable, and the patient will more likely confide in you, and be more adherent to treatment.

The form of the question and the form of the answer

How questions are phrased determines the kind of answer obtained. In over 80% of cases questioning alone is sufficient to enable a diagnosis (Hampton et al, 1975). Two main forms of questions are addressed here: *open* questions ('How are you feeling?') and *closed* questions ('Are you feeling ill?').

The classic example (slightly modified) of how *not* to form a question to a patient:

1. 'Have you stopped beating your husband?'

Notice how this question form traps the patient. The social disapproval in the topic may prevent the patient answering at all. The patient is guilty if they answer yes and guilty if they answer no.

2. 'Are you still having problems with your husband?'

This question is closed because it limits the possible answers to 'yes' or 'no'. It also assumes a problem, and encourages socially desirable answers.

3. 'How's your marriage these days?' or 'How's your husband?' or 'How's the family?'

This more open question form avoids the restrictions of the previous two. Also, these are more general enquiries. What aspect of the marriage? Allowing a range of responses permits the patient to raise the issue of relationship difficulties.

Examples of closed question forms:
- Do you have any pain?
- Do you cough when you lay down?
- Are you worried about your surgery?
- Are you unhappy working on this Unit?
- Did you eat all of your dinner?
- Do you get plenty of exercise?

Examples of open question forms:
- How are things between you and your husband?
- How do you feel?
- What happens if you lie down?
- How do you feel about your forthcoming surgery?
- How do you feel about working with us?
- What did you have for dinner?
- What kinds of exercise do you do?

Notice that closed questions sometimes suggest the answer to the patients, and if they answer randomly, they will be correct 50% of the time. This is not the kind of information to rely on. Also, pressure to answer in a certain socially desirable way can be influential. 'Are you unhappy working on this unit?' carries with it a subtle moral dimension which can reflect badly on the person who answers. This can, and does, bias responses.

Let's look at social desirability more closely. The question form communicates expectancy or preference to the respondent: 'Don't you like it here?'

The question tone as always is important. Emphasis on 'like' and a rising tone on 'here' makes the question rhetorical, imperative, almost indignant if the person questioned isn't happy being 'here'. In contrast, equal emphasis on 'Don't you like' and a lower tone on 'it here' signifies concern, and equal emphasis on all but 'it', which if said in a lower tone may communicate sarcasm.

These three question forms place pressure on the respondent to answer in different ways. But using an open form of this question such as,

'How do you like being here?' or 'Are you settling in?'

also expresses different emphasis, depending on tone, but open questions do not constrain or dictate the preferred answer.

Open questions are mostly used during the early stages of an interview for identifying the range of problems when it is important to avoid suggesting responses to the patient. Of course not all patients, colleagues or co-professionals are going to tell you what they think you want to hear. But in clinical interviews it is desirable to avoid limiting options too early on.

In comparison, closed questions are important in clarifying specific points, such as the timing of events, or the location of pain.

HW: When did this last happen?
Pt: Oh, some time ago now . . . I'm not sure.
HW: Has it happened since Christmas?
Pt: I think so.
HW: Was it more than three months ago?.
Pt: Oh yes.
HW: Did it happen somewhere around June or July time?
Pt: Yes. I think it was during that time.

Generally speaking, open questions provide wider, less specifically directed information and tend to minimize constraints on responses. Closed questions, by comparison, tend to produce directed information often of a constrained form.

Some health workers begin with open questions but progressively use more closed questions to focus the inquiry.

Fact questions: what, where and when

The nature and timing of specific events maybe important to clarify. Previous illness, effective treatments, previous hospitalizations and related reactions may indicate specific interventions. Specific information of this type is required in needs assessment.

Clarification may be needed. Patients sometimes use medical terminology correctly and sometimes incorrectly. Clarify if the respondent is using technical terms correctly. Children and patients with difficulty expressing themselves or with memory problems may need a more careful approach to clarify events.

HW: You said that last time you were in hospital you had a bad reaction to some medicine. How did it affect you?

This open question leaves room for answers ranging from euphoria to anaphylactic shock.

Pt: I felt very dizzy and was all hot and cold.
HW: How long did it last?
Pt: About half an hour, I think.
HW: Could you still walk?
Pt: Yes. The nurse said it often happens with those pills
HW: Do you know what the pills were for?
Pt: I think they were for my water.
HW: Was that the first time you'd had treatment for your water?

The above outline indicates how questioning might proceed. A combination of open and closed questions aids clarification.

HW: How do you feel about the operation tomorrow?
Pt: I'm a bit worried
HW: I understand. How does that make you feel?
Pt: Its on my mind a lot . . . . My stomach's upset.

Using open questions, the nurse identifies how the patient feels about the forthcoming surgery. By clarifying the nature of the patient's worry, the health worker can then apply simple interventions to minimize the worry. Giving reassurance straight away would have overlooked this simple problem. Consider the following exchange:

HW: How did your operation affect you?
Pt: Oh, it helped a lot, but I felt very depressed for weeks afterwards.
HW: What do you mean when you say you felt depressed?
Pt: I couldn't do much and I hate to being looked after. I was sore for quite a while and my young son had been having a difficult time, then when I got home, I still couldn't look after him.
HW: How were you feeling?
Pt: Upset! He was being really naughty. My wife was trying hard to look after both of us and I could tell she was finding it a strain too, even though she didn't say so.
HW: You said you felt 'upset'.
Pt: Yes, I had no appetite. I felt that I had caused everyone a lot of trouble.
HW: Were you feeling guilty?
Pt: Yes, I kept telling myself it was all my fault I'd been ill.

In the above exchange it was important to identify what the patient meant by 'depressed'. The social context of the depression which might influence the patient's acceptance of any future in-patient treatment is potentially important clinical information. A final example illustrates clarification.

HW: Do you have any other problems?
Pt: I get blood pressure now and then.
HW: Blood pressure?
Pt: Yeah.
HW: Does anything happen when you have blood pressure?
Pt: Oh, I get a bad headache.
HW: Tell me about the headache.

Here the blood pressure complained of by the patient may be something else entirely, but would have been overlooked by simply accepting the patient's use of the term.

Location of events such as symptoms may also be important. A similar form of questioning can be used to clarify these.

Asking difficult questions

Sometimes you need to ask about sensitive or embarrassing subjects, something many health workers find difficult. Sexual issues are one area which health workers find particularly difficult to discuss with patients. Topics include contraception; discussing unprotected intercourse with a patient who might be HIV positive; a first pregnancy or a gynecological complaint; functional sexual difficulties; infertility; disorder likely to affect sexual functioning, such as diabetes, multiple sclerosis, or spinal injury; treatments which affect sexual function, such as some anti-hypertensive drugs, psychotropics and diuretics; treatment which affects reproductive function such as anti-cancer chemotherapy; and patients with marital or relationship difficulties.

Many of these topics are among the most common issues patients face. How do we ask about these topics?

If you have established rapport with the patient it is easier to begin. Questions should be unambiguous and both technical and slang terms should be avoided where possible unless this facilitates communication such as when the patient uses the term first. Patients may themselves raise an issue related to sexuality. Some patients may feel embarrassed or have difficulty expressing themselves. A patient may use a common euphemism to avoid difficulties in language, such as:

I can't do it any more.

The health worker should try to clarify the patient's meaning. Reflection is useful

Can't do it any more?

Or rephrase and seek clarification at the same time:

Do you mean you can't have sexual intercourse any more?

The health worker should avoid any suggestion of inadequacy or failure in the patient. It is useful to confirm whether the patient is in a (stable) relationship before asking about sexual activity. An adult can be asked.

Are you married or living with someone?' (Avoid moral judgement.) An adolescent might be asked: 'Do you have a steady boyfriend/girlfriend?'

Instead of asking 'Are you having a sexual problem?', ask 'Do you enjoy sexual activity?' or 'How is your sex life?'

Both open questions avoid implication of problems, but communicate to the patient your interest in and willingness to discuss related topics.

An adolescent or young adult might be asked, 'How do you deal with your sexual feelings?'

For a divorced or widowed patient, the question might be more gently phrased, 'Are you feeling lonely after the death of your spouse?'. Not all relationship problems are sexual.

When exploring functional sexual problems such as erectile difficulty, premature ejaculation, loss of interest in sex, vaginal dryness or orgasmic dysfunction, clear, direct questions are often easiest and most effective.

Do you get erections? How long do they last?
Is sexual intercourse satisfying for you?
Do you still get aroused or excited?
Do you make love as frequently as you would like to?

It is important to ask the patient what their understanding of the problem is.

HW: Is sex satisfying?
Pt: (Shakes head, unhappy look on his face.)
HW: Can you tell me why?

Pt: My wife's not interested any more.

HW: I see. Why do you think that might be?

Pt: Everything was good 'til we had our second child. Since then, though she's always too tired, or there's some other reason.

HW: How old is the child now?

Pt: Eight months.

HW: Does the child sleep well?

Pt: Yes, goes to bed at seven, sleeps till seven the next morning.

HW: Oh, that is good, you're lucky. Is the baby in your room?

Pt: No, he's in his own room.

HW: Have you discussed this with your wife?

Pt: She says she's not interested.

HW: Hmm. So you don't think your wife is tired? She's just giving that as an excuse. Is that it?

Pt: Yes, I get up before her, I work, but she's got plenty of energy to play with the kids, shop and watch the telly all night. Then when it comes to going to bed, she's suddenly too tired.

HW: Why do you think she'd do that?

Pt: I don't know. Say's she doesn't want any more kids and that she's frightened of getting pregnant again.

HW: Do you use contraception?

Pt: The wife doesn't so she expects me to, but it's not as . . . , it's not the same.

HW: Does she know you've come to see me today?

Pt: Yeah, but she thinks it's for my back.

HW: Apart from sex, how's your relationship with your wife?

Pt: Well, it's not too bad. We have arguments, but . . . No, it's all right. We don't go out as much, she's always complaining about that, but money's short, and who looks after the children?

HW: What do you think we should do about it?

This kind of problem is very common and might easily be presented to a general practitioner, for example.

Counselling people about sexual risk is usually most relevant to those aged between 14 and 40 years. Unwanted pregnancy and sexually transmitted diseases are major problems, especially the risk of HIV infection. Counselling may prevent major problems or risk to life and is therefore vitally important for some people. Assuming most young people are increasingly likely to experience intercourse, then it is important to ensure they know how to avoid the risks. A teenage girl wants contraceptive advice from her GP or local family planning clinic. Information and encouraging her to use condoms for contraception and protection from HIV and other sexually transmitted disease might save her life.

Elsewhere, this very important topic can be raised opportunistically in the following manner.

HW: OK. This cream will help to clear up your skin. If it hasn't begun to improve within one week, come back and see me again.

Pt: Thanks.

HW: Miss Chan, could we talk for a moment about something personal, but very important?

Pt: What?

HW: Do you have a boyfriend at the moment?

Pt: Er, yes?

HW: If you are sexually involved, or think you might soon be, there are some important things to consider now.

Pt: What do you mean?

HW: The two biggest problems facing a young woman with normal sexual feelings are unplanned pregnancy and AIDS.

Pt: I don't sleep around you know!

HW: I'm not saying that you do. What I am saying is that when you decide to have sexual intercourse, you need to make sure your partner wears a condom. If you do, you will reduce your risk of AIDS and pregnancy very much.

Pt: OK.

HW: I realize that this wasn't something that you came here to find out, but even the nicest people get pregnant or catch the AIDS virus. I make it a habit to tell as many people as I can. I hope you don't mind?

Pt: No, no. Thanks. Uhm . . .

(Pause.)

HW: Yes?

Pt: My friend's boyfriend won't wear one.

HW: How does she feel about that?

Pt: She's worried that if she makes him, he'll leave her.

HW: That can be a problem. Some boys think it's the woman's responsibility to stop getting pregnant. But your friend's boyfriend needs to consider that a condom will not just protect her, it will help protect him too.

Pt: She likes him a lot.

HW: I can see it's difficult for her. But a condom could protect her from AIDS. That must be more important. Talk to her about it. You might do her a big favour.

Pt: Yeah.

So sensitive topics can be raised without difficulty, despite the presenting problem being completely unrelated. The health education role of the practitioner warrants such discussion.

Feeling questions: feelings, then and now

Health workers, particularly students, find difficulty in dealing with patients' feelings. Studies indicate this is a major area of anxiety for most health care students. There is little reason to believe this changes substantially after graduation. Eliciting feelings and responding to emotive questions is an important set of skills for the health worker to acquire, particularly medical practitioners, psychiatric and community nurses, hospice staff, speech therapists, counsellors and psychologists.

The term 'feeling' can be used to elicit a broad range of responses. For example, clarifying feelings is particularly important in a psychosocial interview; in assessing the impact of a procedure or treatment; in interactions with children or patients with serious, life threatening or disabling conditions and in chronic pain states.

Eliciting feelings, identifying them and relating them to different circumstances can be very helpful in adaptation and coping within health care settings.

Four simple strategies that can be used are:
- asking about current feelings
- asking about past feelings
- asking patients to recall a situation that evoked a similar feeling
- asking patients to describe the parts of their body affected by feelings

Patients need to be willing to discuss feelings. Not all patients are willing or able to do so. If patients do not want to discuss feelings, the health worker might gently explore the reasons why.

Patients who find it difficult to describe their feelings can be encouraged to use whatever metaphors to help them to express themselves. Resorting to other techniques, such as asking them to write down descriptions or drama, may be tried but are seldom practical in general health care setting.

Some patients have great difficulty in identifying feelings, sometimes called *alexithymia* (literally, no words for feelings). More careful and specialist help may be needed with such patients. With these exceptions, most patients are able and willing to discuss feelings. Eliciting feelings can be a simple task, but one that requires sensitivity and consideration.

Asking about current feelings

The most obvious way to elicit information on patients' feelings is to ask directly. The health worker should avoid suggesting how the patient might feel at first, though this may be tried if the patient needs some help. Be careful after suggesting responses that the patient doesn't simply repeat them back.

HW: How do you feel about coming into hospital?
Pt: It's better than being dead.
HW: That doesn't sound very optimistic.
Pt: Well, I'm not overjoyed about it. It interferes with my work.
HW: It sounds like you're annoyed about that.
Pt: I am. I was hoping to start a new project. We'd just got a contract and I was really looking forward to doing it. And then this had to happen.
HW: How do you feel inside?
Pt: Pretty angry because someone else will be given the project that I put all the work into.

Note how the health worker perceives the patient, 'It sounds like you're annoyed . . .'. This can be a particularly useful tool to facilitate patients' talking about their feelings. Very often, when feelings are discussed, they become more intense, enabling the person to also vent much feeling. This can help to make patients feel better afterwards, though sometimes they may feel worse, if the feeling is upsetting for them.

Asking about past feelings

A similar approach works well for eliciting past feelings, but with an added dimension in that you can ask patients how they feel about the event in retrospect, and this may add further to the value of the discussion.

HW: How did you feel when you were told you had to have your toes amputated?
Pt: Awful. I didn't expect that it would, you know, happen to me, like. I was really depressed for about three or four weeks after the operation. I kept thinking, what will they chop off next?
HW: You said you were depressed. How did that make you feel?
Pt: Well, I couldn't put my mind to anything. I had no interest in anything, and I, ah, I just couldn't see anything to look forward

to, even though my daughter was pregnant with her first child at the time.

HW: What else?

Pt: I lost my appetite. I just sat around at home all day feeling miserable.

HW: Miserable?

Pt: Yeah, weepy and down, like there was no future anymore. I felt like it was, you know, like the first step to the grave.

HW: It sounds like you felt pretty bad.

Pt: Yeah.

HW: Looking back at that time, do you feel the same way about it now?

Pt: No, not now. I mean you can't stay like that can you? After I was up and about, the wife kept on at me to see the doctor again, but there's nothing he could do, is there? No, I think you've just got to keep going as best you can. . . .that's all.

(Pause.)

Pt: I'll tell you something, though, I wish there was some way of getting me toes back.

HW: You still miss them, do you? . . . etc.

A mixture of techniques are used here. Clarification of the term depressed, reflection ('Miserable?') and empathic statements all help to explore the patient's mood and feelings. The health worker elicited and discussed how the patient felt without discomfort to either.

Asking patients to recall a situation that evoked a similar feeling

Asking patients directly may be unsuccessful, especially with children who may be unable to respond to the abstract labels we give to feelings. This approach asks the patient to recall or describe a situation that evokes similar feelings.

HW: Let's try a different way. Can you think of a time or something that happened that made you feel the same way as you feel now?

Pt: When I was a child . . .

HW: Perhaps.

Pt: I, I sometimes would fight with my parents, and . . . they usually ended with, ah, with me being punished. Afterwards, I used to feel . . . I don't know, this sounds silly, but I used to think I was on fire inside. I wasn't hot, but it was like I imagined, you know, it would feel like.

HW: Do you feel like that now?

Pt: Not really, but it's the nearest I can think of, like everything was on fire, or something.

HW: Could you think of a situation you think might make you, or someone else feel like you do now?

Pt: Er. . . . that's quite hard. Maybe if you were, you know, if you couldn't breathe. You know how it feels like when you can't breathe and you want to, like if you're underwater or something. I don't know, that's . . . that's the only thing . . .

HW: So its maybe like a cross between not being able to breath and feeling like there's a fire inside you?

Pt: Yeah, I suppose . . . like there's a fire in your stomach and you can't breathe any air, but it doesn't burn, just makes you feel like you're very hot. And I, I can't think clearly then, I just want to get away . . .

Here an imaginary situation helped the patient fill in the bits that the past event didn't provide. The patient is then presented with this 'collage' by the health worker, and is able to add on bits to make a fuller picture of current feelings. The important thing is not to describe the feelings but to identify what they mean for the patient. Thus, the patient at the end says, 'I can't think clearly, and I just want to get away . . .' Specialist input may be needed but the health worker has clarified what is being experienced. Thus it becomes more understandable, and hence more controllable. This can help make it less stressful for the patient.

Asking patients to describe the parts of their body affected by feelings

Helping people localize, where possible, their feelings in their body may help with understanding them. Some feelings may be associated with the stomach, others seem to affect the heart or lungs. Some people can localize their feelings better than others, so not everybody can benefit from this technique.

HW: Does the feeling seem to affect or be felt in any particular part of your body?

Pt: Well, my heart seems like it's going to jump out of my chest, it's pounding so fast, and my mouth seems really dry as well.

HW: Hmmm. Do you feel it anywhere else?

Pt: In the pit of my stomach, like . . . like, I want to go to the toilet, or something like that.

This technique is simple and, with sensitivity, can be used very effectively. It may be especially useful if the patient is talking about traumatic events, for example, accidental burns, road accidents, bereavement and bad news situations.

Closing the interview

Closing an interview well is as important as to begin it well. The end of an interview has three distinct sections. First, *check* the information given by the patient has been clearly understood, or that the issue under discussion can be left. Second, *inquire* if the patient has anything further to add or any questions. Third, make a clear *closing statement*.

Check the information

This involves briefly summarizing the main points, and asking if there is anything that has been left out.

HW: So it seems then that the main problems are first your leg, second, the problems you've been having with your child, and third, the money side of things. Are they the main points?
Pt: Yeas, that and my diabetes.
HW: Yes, I'm sure it's your diabetes that is causing your leg problems. Is there anything I've missed out?

Where the discussion of an unresolved problem has to be discontinued, something along the following lines is appropriate;

HW: So what is going to happen now?
Pt: Well, I suppose I have to try and come to terms with it, but . . . I don't know . . .
HW: Hmmm. I can see you still aren't very sure. Why don't we leave there for now? You think about what we've discussed and we'll talk some more tomorrow. Does that sound alright?
Pt: OK.

Anything more to add?

Checking if the patient has any more to add can be simply carried out.

> Is there anything else before we finish?
> Do you have anything to add to what we've discussed?
> Anything else?

and most importantly;

> Do you have any questions?
> Is there anything you'd like to know before we finish?

Closing statement

The clear concluding statement can be similarly brief.

> If that's okay we can stop here. I'll see you again tomorrow.
> If that's all, we'll end there for now.
> Well, this seems like a good place to break off for now.

The benefit of ending the interview positively lies in the clear, mutually agreed (usually) decision that the interview is over. Failure to do this can leave patients, and even staff uncertain if an interview will re-commence, or if a temporary absence means the interview is over, and so forth.

Confidentiality

As with other patient information, appropriate levels of confidentiality need to be maintained. Confidentiality is less than perfect in most hospitals. Case notes contain a wide range of information. The increase in psychosocial history taking means that sensitive information is also collected. The question then arises about what to do with such information.

For example, does a GP who learns that a patient's husband visits a prostitute regularly make a note of this in the medical record? Should this information be passed on to the patient who might be at increased risk of AIDS as a result of her husband's activity? This presents an ethical dilemma which is difficult to resolve.

What if a patient is an employee of the hospital wherein she is a patient? What information goes into her case notes, which will almost certainly be read by some of her colleagues? What if it emerges that she is an illicit drug user? What if she is HIV positive yet remains well? How can this patient's confidentiality be protected?

The disposal of information given by patients remains largely unresolved, despite the brief emergence of the dilemma about ten years ago. There appears to be no clear solution other than maintaining confidentiality wherever possible. There are situations where this is impossible with traditional written medical records. Clearly, some different means of recording patient data need to be developed. This issue is discussed further in Chapter 13.

Summary

- Maintain attention to patients when they are talking.
- When you are talking, the patient cannot speak.
- Talk less, listen more.
- Listen for verbal cues as the patient is talking, specifically:
  - emotional content
  - pauses
  - unwillingness to answer questions
  - stuttering
  - changes in tone of voice/voice tension
- Clarify technical terms, e.g. depressed, hypertension, etc. when used by patients; they may mean something different.
- Establish goals for treatment with the patient's participation; most people want to be involved in treatment decision making, not just be medicine receptacles.
- Watch the patients as they speak; look for non-verbal cues.
- Remember that you will also be giving cues to the patient; therefore be:
  - accepting
  - non-judgemental
  - warm
- Use open questions to identify areas of focus, or when talking about psychological aspects of the patient.
- Use closed questions to narrow down the area of questioning.
- When asking questions about factual events, allow the patient to explain.
- Questions on sexual matters should be clear and reasonably direct.
- Discussing feelings needs sensitivity.

- Use empathic statements, such as:
  - asking about current feelings
  - asking about past feelings
  - asking patients to recall a situation that evoked a similar feeling
  - asking patients to describe the parts of their body affected by feelings
- End the interview by:
  - summarizing and checking information
  - asking if there is anything to add
  - asking if the patient has any questions
  - making a clear concluding statement

Exercises

1. Interviewer: the task is to ask the interviewees about one event in their lives that has significance for them. Practise using open and closed question forms. Make use of verbal and non-verbal cues to try and identify any emotional elements of the event. Do not question the interviewees directly on their feelings. Instead use empathic statements to identify any feeling. Spend 5 to 20 minutes. Afterwards, discuss the feelings experienced by the interviewees and compare. Exchange roles.

2. Health worker and patient. Negotiate the goals and degree of involvement the 'patients' would want if they were diagnosed as having cancer, cardiovascular disease, renal disease, or muscular/joint disease. Practise open and closed question forms. How much involvement is expected, and why do the 'patients' want that. How would they feel if this was denied them, or if the opportunity was never presented for participation in goal planning? Spend 5 to 10 minutes. Change roles and compare.

3. Question the interviewee on an emotional event in interviewee's life. Use emotion questioning techniques, open/closed questions and empathic statements. Spend 15 to 20 minutes exploring the feelings of the interviewee. Change roles. Give feedback on interviewer's performance.

Discussion

1. To what extent should the health worker take time to identify the patient's feelings about treatments/diagnoses having implications for survival? For example, if the patient has cancer, should the patient's feelings about treatment have priority over all other decisions?

2. How much can health workers expect patients to be honest with information? Consider the case of a patient who tests positive for HIV.

3. To what extent should doctors, nurses and other health professionals be responsible for dealing with patients' emotional responses to their situation?

7

Guiding the Interview

Educational Objectives

By the end of this chapter, you should be able to

- outline the main components of negotiation
- demonstrate an effective negotiation technique
- demonstrate an adequate level of control over a clinical interview
- list further reasons for the involvement of the patient in decision making
- give further details of techniques for negotiating the patient's level of involvement
- list reasons why patients may wonder off the point during interview
- give examples of how to re-direct a patient back to the topic in hand
- recognize the role of precision in information giving as an aid to focus the patient
- recognize the role of cross-checking
- identify ways to identify uncertainty or mis-understanding in the patient
- describe the purpose of clarifying uncertainties
- recognize the effects of closed questioning with untalkative clients
- list techniques for handling talkative patients

Introduction

How much should the health worker control and direct the interview? How much control should the patient/client/staff member being interviewed be given? How much control the health worker exerts or allows the patient will depend upon the purpose and goals of the interviewer and interviewee — the participants.

We know many non-biological problems that people take to their doctors are not identified. At one time, patients commonly complained that many doctors decided treatment before the consultation began. The prescription form on the doctor's desk would be completed with the exception of the name of the medication to be prescribed. Conversely, many patients expect or demand some form of tangible treatment from the consultation. Unfortunately there is clear evidence that the provision of prescription drugs has been abused at the cost of better communications to identify underlying reasons for consultation (Cochrane, 1972; Hayward, 1975).

Similarly, admission or discharge interviews in hospitals often focus on a few distinct areas: medication, follow-up appointments, do's and don't's. It is still the exception rather than the rule for discharge interviews to involve patients.

In most interviews, GP or specialist consultations, admission and discharge interviews, the patient is likely to have different goals to the health worker. These may include questions on treatment efficacy, side effects of medication, returning to work, and other more psychosocial-oriented information (Fielding, 1987). Often this information is either not provided or given in such a way that patients fail to recall it (Ley, 1982). Also the clinical interview gives little opportunity for patients to introduce their own material, unless the normal progress of the interview is overridden by interjecting information or questions (Drass, 1982). Even then these may be ignored by health workers intent on getting their facts. Alternatively, the health worker can negotiate with the patient the format of the interview, perhaps agreeing to deal with the patient's inquiries first, then giving additional information not covered by the patient's questions. Considering the patient's needs for the interview and how negotiation and control may be carried out to best effect is addressed in the remainder of this section.

Negotiating the topic for discussion

Why should the health worker take the time and trouble to meet the patient's appropriate goals of the consultation? Generally, the advantages

gained in meeting the patient's needs relate to improved patient evaluation of treatment (Buller and Buller, 1988), greater patient satisfaction
(Korsch and Negrete 1972), and better recall of, and adherence with
medical recommendations (Ley, 1988; Michembaum and Turk, 1987).
(See Chapters 1, 5 and 6.)

Where no goal has been negotiated between the health worker and
the patient, each may have different expectations of the nature of an
interview. For example, consider the traditional stereotype format of an
out-patient consultation described by Drass (1982) and outlined in Chapter
5. Under conditions that might better be described as a cross-examination,
the patient is usually offered little involvement either in deciding the
direction of the interview, or any responsibility for the outcome. Not
surprisingly patient satisfaction with such consultations is low, and
adherence with subsequent treatment poor.

A wide range of examples has demonstrated one consistent principle:
when people participate in creating something, they have more interest in
preserving it than if they passively receive it.

Szasz and Hollender (1956) identify three distinct types of doctor–
patient relationship. These typologies also apply to other health – patient
relationships. The relationships so far described in the present chapter
constitute the 'guidance – cooperation' type. Here the patient is cooperative with the health worker's guidance. At times when the patient might
be unconscious, as during an operation, the 'activity – passivity' type of
relationship is said to exist. Here, the health worker is active, the patient
however, totally passive. The third form of relationship proposed by
Szasz and Hollender (1956) takes the form of 'mutual participation'.

The need to include patients in their own health care has been previously described (Szasz and Hollender, 1956; Brody, 1980; Turk and
Meichenbaum, 1987). Patients need to be active participants in the health
care process, both in terms of decision making (Meichenbaum and Turk,
1987) and in terms of therapeutics (Anderson and Kirk, 1982). As
Meichenbaum and Turk (1987) pointed out,

> A call for such active participation does not in any way compro-
> mise the expertise of the health worker in the examination and
> diagnosis of the patient's presenting clinical problems, but instead
> it underscores the underlying equality between health worker's
> and patient's responsibilities for the outcome of treatment.

Patients who become actively involved in their own care demonstrate
a more favourable outcome (Schulman, 1979), with greater patient satisfaction (Eisenthal, Emory, Lazare and Udin, 1979), than patients not so
involved.

Most research shows that as people are expected to do more to care for their own health, such as modify lifestyle habits, most patients fail repeatedly to change their health behaviour. Increasing the knowledge of patients is not in itself sufficient to lead to changed health behaviour. If only knowledge was needed to change health behaviour, no one would smoke tobacco or have unprotected intercourse. So, while information is probably a necessary component of behaviour change, it is not an adequate component for such change. Involvement in decision making also gives more responsibility to patients for their own well-being. This involvement stimulates interest making task success more likely. Encouraging patient involvement in decision making is therefore beneficial to both the health worker and patient.

Technique: negotiating goals

How is negotiation achieved? Some basic suggestions can be found in Chapter 5. Remember, begin the negotiation process with an open question form, even if there appears to be an obvious cause for consultation. Do not assume this is the (only) reason why the patient is consulting.

Seek indications from the patient using open questions.
e.g.

> Hello Mrs Young. What can I do for you?
> Good morning Mr Lee. What brings you here today?

If the patient has come for a follow-up appointment, or is in hospital and is approached by the health worker you might say the following:
e.g.

HW: Well, thank you for coming today Mr Lee. As you may remember, we asked you to come to see how you are managing with your new treatment. How have you been managing?

or,

HW: Good Morning Mrs Chan. I'm Nurse/Dr Lee, and I'm taking care of you while you're here. How are you?

Pt: Okay.

HW: Good. Now, there are some tests that we need to do today, which I'll tell you about in a minute. But before I do, is there anything that you would like us to look at for you while you are here?

Pt: My eyes are very bad, and my glasses don't work well any more. Can you do something?

In this last example, the patient may have been admitted for some minor surgery, for example, and asks the health worker to 'do something' about her eyes. This needs clarification. Where the deterioration is due to normal changes, it may be inappropriate or not really that particular health worker's area to deal with opthalmics, and if no referral can practically be made, it might be quite acceptable to say so.

HW: Well, Mrs Chan, I've had a quick look, and I can't see anything. Its likely that you need new glasses. You should have your eyes tested when you go home. We can't test your eyes here. I will also mention this in my letter to your GP. He can then follow it up. Is there anything else you think we might help with?

Pt: No, I don't think so. What tests are you going to do?

HW: Well, shall I tell you what we have in mind, and if you agree to that we can get on and you should be home for the weekend. Does that sound alright?

Perhaps the patient requests medication that is not really needed:

HW: Hello Mr Lee, What can I do for you?

Pt: It's my back again doctor. Can you give me something to put it right? It's a real problem.

HW: I see. Well, let's see, last time you came we sent you for some physical therapy. Didn't that help?

Pt: Yes, a bit. But . . . its still very painful.

HW: (nods)

Pt: I think I need something stronger for the pain.

HW: I'd like to have someone else look at your back if you don't mind? I think we need to know precisely what the trouble is before we decide what to do.

Pt: Alright, but can you give me something in the meantime?

HW: You've been taking the pain-killer I gave you last time?

Pt: Yes, but . . . I think I need something stronger.

HW: Hmm. Well, I think we should look closely at what you are doing to make your back easier. I don't know that just giving you stronger pain-killers is the best answer. There are several other things we might try such as physiotherapy, relaxation and maybe some massage. Then we can decide on how best we can manage your back problem. I think we might be able to sort it out better, rather than simply giving you some pills and sending you off again. And we'll look at your medication too.

Pt: Well, okay.

The health worker may have to be more direct in addressing the patient — in this case about the management of chronic back pain — while still using negotiation. The patient's expectations of consultation may sometimes be wholly inappropriate or unrealistic. If so, rather than dismissing out of hand the patient's expectations, educating them about the inappropriateness or ineffectiveness of their wishes is the best approach.

Key Points

Negotiation is important. It increases the chance that a health worker will address the patient's concerns, improving patient satisfaction, and sense of involvement and responsibility for the patient's health. Also, the health worker is more likely to achieve cooperation and adherence to treatment if this is the case.

As a result both patient and practitioner are likely to be more satisfied with the consultation.

Negotiating goals with children

It is also necessary to negotiate with children about treatment and adherence, but to a lesser extent about interview goals. With young children it is usually the parent who makes the decision to seek a medical opinion. The child often has little say in the decision to consult, and (sometimes) tends to remain passive throughout the interview.

Older children, when given the opportunity to consult independently of their parents, demonstrate appropriate help-seeking behaviour. Adolescents, particularly those over sixteen, are increasingly likely to consult their doctor alone. With older adolescents, an adult approach is appropriate. In younger adolescents and older children, the health worker may negotiate with the patient, more with an educational intent to encourage the growing person to adopt more responsibility for his or her health. In most cases, young children often willingly accede to a health worker's recommendations for the interview aims, but it is good for the patient to be encouraged to participate from an early age.

◼ Keeping to the agreed topic

Once the topic/focus of the interview has been agreed, the most common remaining problem is probably keeping to the topic. The patient may talk about something which the health worker does not think relevant. There may be a need to bring the patient back to the topic in hand. However, it is important to be aware that this may be an attempt by the patient to introduce new material relevant to the discussion. This can be checked by the following.

HW: How is that important for your present problem?

It is quite possible that this other business is the real reason for the patient's visit. If this is dismissed, it may reinforce the patient's anxiety that the problem is not appropriate to consult a practitioner about. It may also mean the practitioner overlooks potentially important information.

Other problems include patients who find it difficult in expressing themselves or who are unwilling to talk for a variety of reasons, health workers who might be more at home in a interrogation chamber than a clinic, and health workers who dream they are on the golf course during an interview.

One reason why patients may wander off the point is their uncertainty about what information the health worker wants. So, by clarifying what information is sought patients may be helped to provide more focused information.

HW: How does your stomach feel after you have not eaten for a while. Does that affect you?

Technique

Keeping to the topic is in most cases managed by the use of a few choice statements which serve to redirect the patient back to the topic in hand. e.g.

        Do you see that as important to your being unwell?
        Does/did that affect your present illness?
        If you don't think that is too important to your present illness, could we look more at you present problem. When exactly did the pain begin?

or,

        Can we get back to your present illness?

or,

> That must have been annoying, but to return to your pain . . . .
> when exactly did it begin?

Encouraging relevance is useful and is achieved by encouraging precision where possible regarding dates of symptoms, problems or events, previous treatments, and so forth. The cross checking of points is also useful and helps to maintain relevance and accuracy at the same time.

> You said you live with your family. Who lives at your house?

The clarification of uncertainties can be used to regain relevance in an interview.

> Sorry. I'm unsure about what your work involves. Can we talk
> about that?

What follows are a series of specific problems that may occur from time to time with suggestions for dealing with these.

Untalkative patients

Adults

Some patients have difficulty in expressing themselves. Children, adolescents, persons with psychosexual problems, participants or victims of intra-familial abuse, torture, rape or other forms of violence, may not talk for different reasons. Cultural prohibitions limit discussion of certain topics, for example sexual behaviour, and the health worker may also be bound by the same prohibitions. Encouraging conversation is thus an important skill.

It is understandable that a patient may be unwilling to talk or discuss intimate personal topics where privacy or confidentiality cannot be guaranteed. So, trying to take a psychosexual history from a patient in a crowded ward is not likely to be very successful, and cause discomfort or embarrassment to the patient. Find a side room or somewhere where the patient feels secure that the conversation will not be overheard. A simple, but often overlooked remedy, particularly in places where crowding is the norm.

Inform the patient in advance that you would like to discuss a sensitive topic. This can sometimes give the patient time to think of ways of expression.

HW: Hello Mrs Lee. How are you feeling today?

Pt: I am fine, thank you.

HW: Was your husband not able to be here today?

Pt: He has to work.

HW: Mrs Lee, as I explained in my letter to you, I need to ask you some questions about your sexual relationship with your husband if I am to understand why you have not yet had children. Is that alright?

Pt: (Avoids eye contact, looks at floor, nods slightly.)

HW: Can we begin by you telling me, do you and your husband sleep together?

Pt: (Nods slightly.)

HW: Do you have your own bedroom?

Pt: Yes.

HW: Who else lives with you?

Pt: My husband's mother and father and younger brother.

HW: Do you have privacy? . . . etc.

Note how negotiation of the patient's agreement to discuss or answer questions on sensitive issues helped after the health worker took the trouble to explain to the patient the need for the information. This may help achieve patient cooperation.

There is a distinction to be made between handling patients who don't talk because they are embarrassed or are unwilling to, and those who don't talk because they don't know what to say. It can be particularly difficult to deal with this problem if the patient is not motivated to help the health worker. However, this is not very common; most patients cooperate to resolve their problems. Hence, patients may not be untalkative so much as unable to find words to express themselves.

The following exchange illustrates one way that such patients may be assisted:

HW: Is your headache made worse by anything?

Pt: I don't know.

HW: Well, have you noticed the headache worsen after eating certain foods, for example?

Pt: I don't know.

HW: When is your headache worst?

Pt: Usually at night, I think.

HW: Before you go to bed?

Pt: Yes. Sometimes I can't sleep. It's so bad.

HW: Does it ever wake you up at night?

Pt: Sometimes.

HW: Often?
Pt: No.
HW: Do you drink alcohol with your evening meal or after?
Pt: Sometimes I drink wine.
HW: What colour?
Pt: Red mostly . . . . etc

The health worker is having to ask a mixture of small and careful questions, both open and closed, to find the required answers without suggesting to the patient what this answer should be. This is laborious but reduces the chances of the patient responding 'yes' simply to please the health worker.

Sometimes, a different approach to helping patients express them-selves may be required. (See also Chapter 6.)

HW: How are you feeling today?
Pt: Okay.
HW: I imagine you must have lots of things on your mind after talking with the doctor yesterday.
Pt: (Does not respond.)
HW: It must have been quite a shock . . .
Pt: I still can't believe it. I never thought it would happen to me.
HW: It's hard to deal with.
Pt: I don't know what to do for the best.
HW: Would it help to talk about it now?

Where patients are embarrassed, they may feel easier talking to some-one else, possibly a member of their own, or the opposite sex, someone younger or someone older, or the same age as themselves.

HW: I'd like to ask about your sexual activities.
Pt: I . . . uhm . . . (Looks away.)

(Pause.)

HW: I can see this is difficult for you, but it is important I ask you about this.
Pt: Er . . . . yes.

(Pause.)

HW: If it would it be easier I can ask one of our male nurses to talk with you if you'd prefer?
Pt: I think it would be easier.

HW: Okay. We'll just clear up some other details then I'll ask someone else to come over to talk with you. Is that alright?

Don't use this approach to simply avoid dealing with difficult subjects. Also a bit of forethought can help avoid this sort of embarrassment, such as having a nurse the same gender as the patient do psychosexual interviews. If the health worker is more embarrassed than the patient, then the health worker may need to talk with someone to help overcome any embarrassment.

Where patients may be unwilling to talk about a topic, and it is necessary for information to be gathered on that topic, a process of persuasion may be required.

HW: Are you married, Mr Lee?
Pt: No, . . . I'm not.
HW: Do you have a close friend?
Pt: I don't see why that's important.
HW: Well, the reason I ask is because we like to know if there is anyone to support you. As you have no family, you may be on your own.
Pt: There is someone.
HW: Are they supportive to you?
Pt: Not really. Look, do we have to talk about this?
HW: I can see that you don't want to discuss this. Is there a particular reason that it is difficult?
Pt: Yes, there is; I don't think it's relevant.
HW: I see. Perhaps if I explain why it's relevant it will help. We need to plan your care. You are going to need care after discharge. We need to know who can help because they will need to be taught what to do. We don't have to deal with it now, but please think about it.

The patient clearly did not want to discuss the questions that the health worker raised at this time. It may be necessary to return to the topic at a later time.

Sometimes patients may have impaired language or hearing. Patients who may have partially or totally lost expressive or receptive language after a stroke still need communication. More so, for what has been lost is felt most acutely. Whereas stroke patients may not be able to answer questions or may only partially respond, it is important to continue to explain to such patients what procedures are to be carried out. Lack of expressive communication does not exclude the patient understanding what is said. Where there is suspicion or evidence of loss of language function, physical contact can provide some communication of concern and caring. Specialist assessment of language function will help to plan communication approaches with language-disabled stroke patients.

Patients who are hearing or speech impaired may need special consideration. Each major hospital should have at least one clinical communications expert who is able to use sign language.

Children and adolescents

Children and adolescents require a somewhat different approach. Many children aged less than five years old are uncommunicative due to anxiety or embarrassment. Pressuring the child will further increase the level of anxiety. Anxiety in children under five years old is likely to be related to either fear of separation from the main caretaker; fear of pain (injections, etc.); or previous unpleasant experiences with health care.

So the following arrangements need to be made prior to interviewing a young child:

1. Ensure the main caretaker is present and that the child feels secure with this person. If the child does not feel secure with the caretaker, is there someone else the child feels secure with?
2. If the child refuses to reply, find out from the child or caretaker any past contact and experiences with health care. This will help to identify events which may have sensitized the child to health workers. Cross check the caretaker's evaluations with the child, as in the following example:

HW: (To the four-year-old child) Have you ever been in hospital before?
Pt: (Withdraws closer to mother.)
Mo: About nine months ago. He had a high fever. The doctor wanted him in hospital. But he was alright, came home two days later, didn't you, Tim?
HW: Did you like being in hospital, Tim?
Pt: (Buries face in mother.)
Mo: He was a bit upset because I couldn't stay with him. I'd just had a baby and was feeding her myself.
HW: (To child) That must have been scary!
Pt: (No response.)
HW: I expect you don't like hospitals and doctors and nurses after that?
Pt: (Shakes head.)
HW: Do you think the same thing will happen this time?
Pt: (Nods slightly.)

HW: Well, there's is no need for you to come in to hospital this time. You will be at home with your mum. But would you come to see me here?

Pt: (Nods slightly.)

3. Avoid wearing white coat/uniform. Try to arrange for the clinic, consulting or interview room to have some toys and decorations suitable for children of this age group. By making the visit a more enjoyable experience, you will help overcome any previous negative consequences arising from earlier experiences with health care. Patience may be needed. With older children assurance that all you want to do is spend some time talking and that there will be no injections or other things done to them just now (if that is the case).

Empathy is always beneficial with young children, though empathy alone may not be enough to get them to talk. Other reasons to consider for non-communicativeness in young children are shyness and lack of understanding.

Shyness has no easy solution beyond getting to know the child a bit more. There is no shortcut to this, but spending time playing with the child should help to familiarize the child with the health worker and help overcome shyness. Building rapport is very important if there is to be prolonged contact between doctor and child.

Lack of understanding can confuse a child. Health workers often fail to consider children's level of intellectual development and familiarity with their body. A child may have concepts of health and illness which vary markedly from those of the health worker. It is important for the health worker to explore these. (See Chapter 3.)

For a school-age child (over five years of age), follow the same approach as for younger children. However, older children who do not speak may be significantly more anxious, shy or traumatized. Alternatively, they may be in the health facility against their will. It is important to clarify the reasons for the child's reticence. Again, anxiety is a frequent reason. Older children can be very aware of the social stigma attached to illness, and it is very important to them not to be considered different by their peers. This may be a reason for uncooperativeness or unwillingness to attend. If so, this will need to be dealt with.

Adolescents may be able to express why they are unwilling to cooperate much more and a combination of techniques useful for an older child and young adult would be appropriate.

Talkative patients

Encouraging patients to speak may be problematic, but so is guiding talkative patients to focus on the topic in question and to be concise. Remember the style of the question often determines the style of the answer.

Vague or general questions often elicit vague and general responses. A more precise question may help restrict the scope of the answer. Where patients will not keep to the point it may be necessary to use more controlling or directive strategies to achieve the purposes of the interview. Check that the patient is not trying to raise relevant information. If not, an assertive approach which often works is to ignore the patient's irrelevant answers. If the patient continues to deviate from the question, it may be necessary to point out to the patient that time is limited and unless the answers are direct the health worker won't be able to help.

Children are usually direct. However, young children may tend to give affirmative answers to the *structure* of the question used rather than the question content and the health worker needs to be very cautious in choosing appropriate question formats that are both age appropriate and considered.

The interrogator

Health workers who interrogate patients and get information by virtual intimidation rarely perceive many problems with their communication style. However, they may perceive they have many more 'problem' patients who don't or won't follow treatment recommendations, or worse. Over-control during interviews is a problem for such health workers. There may be several reasons for such an interaction style, but it is beyond the scope of this text to consider them here.

Over-control seldom gets good results compared to a negotiated and shared strategy. Most patients respond best to mutual participation which treats all patients as unique, thus allowing the health worker–patient dyad to develop the most suitable interaction style. This in turn facilitates exchange and enables an approach not reliant on control.

Different stages of the interaction require differing amounts of guidance. Sensitivity to when control is not needed is important. Children often do not respond positively to a controlling approach. Young children are likely to feel intimidated and frightened and may become uncooperative as their only means of expressing their objection to being controlled. This will impair any trust the health worker may hope to develop. Adolescents may be better managed as young adults. Avoid treating them like children which, in their eyes, they no longer are.

The fly-on-the-wall

Another problem during interview is where insufficient control over the interview is maintained so that it becomes directionless. An unwillingness to interrupt or direct the patient to relevant areas causes problems. Some patients will tell you all their family history, beginning with their great grandparent's birth problems. It is worth remembering that the patient, unless given very clear guidelines before you ask them to talk, will not always know what information you need.

There is an important distinction to be made between periodic control or direction, and the total absence of any involvement. Such lack of involvement may occur when a health worker is interacting with more than one individual, such as a husband and wife, or a parent and child.

An example of this was seen in a consultation by a mother and her two young sons. The two boys had sore throats. The trainee practitioner was clearly unsure what information to gather and both children quickly began to ignore the health worker and explored the office. The health worker asked one or two questions from the mother. But feeling control was slipping away, the health worker was left speechless, watching the growing chaos in the office. The children and the mother became very restless, waiting for the health worker to take control, which was never done. Needless to say, the consultation was not successful.

More control is needed under such circumstances, and it would have been appropriate to ask the children directly to sit down, or the mother to keep her sons seated if they refuse.

Key Points

Appropriate levels of control are necessary throughout an interview or interaction. The degree or extent that the health worker exercises control over different aspects of the interaction: the questioning, the relevance of the answers, the pacing of the interaction (timing), and the degree of involvement are a major dimension of the interaction. Too much or too little control can inhibit the exchange.

Summary

Negotiate goals for each interaction with patient
- Use open question forms for negotiation
- Check that the patient agrees with the goals before proceeding

Help the patient keep to the agreed topic by:
- emphasizing relevance in answering questions
- emphasizing precision with dates, etc.
- cross checking points with the patient
- clarifying uncertainties
- ensuring the patient knows what information you are interested in

Exercises

Take about five minutes before beginning the role play to read through the roles and familiarize yourself with the parts and the tasks.

1. *Situation:* The location is a general ward in a busy hospital. The patient has chronic asthma and was admitted following an acute episode. The health worker is going to take a history of the patient's previous hospital experience.
    Time available: 7 minutes.

    You are the patient. (Be your own age.) You are indistinct about details when asked. You have suffered from asthma since you were very young, and have been hospitalized many times. You are in hospital now following yet another attack of asthma. You know that in two or three days, you will be discharged once more and are fed up with all of the questions you are asked. Every time you come into hospital with asthma you face the same questions. You are fed up of questions and want more concrete help.

2. *Situation:* In an out-patient clinic or health centre, the health worker is taking the history of a patient — a 32-year-old mother of two.

    You are the patient. Your four-year-old daughter is always getting colds and flu. Your seven-year-old son was diagnosed nine months ago as having juvenile diabetes mellitus. So far he has been well, but you have felt increasingly tired and have frequent headaches. Your children take most of your time.

If asked about your headaches or tiredness, be unsure about the times and dates. Keep returning to the topic of your oldest son's ability to lead a normal life, adaptation to insulin injections, etc and seek reassurance from the health worker for his health, and the health of your daughter. Keep changing the subject.

3. *Situation:* A young, single adult is visiting an out-patient clinic for the first time. The patient complains of fatigue, loss of weight and a persistent dry cough. The health worker suspects HIV infection (AIDS or AIDS related complex). The health worker needs to find out if the patient uses or has used intravenous drugs, and details of the patient's sexual activities over the last year.

You are the patient. You have been losing weight, feeling tired and have a persistent dry cough for about ten weeks. (Be vague about how long and details.) You either:
(a) used intravenous drugs only once about 18 months ago, to see what it was like (knowing that the needle was new and unused). You have not been sexually active during the last two years. If asked about drug-taking change the subject. Talk about your cough.
or
(b) You have been sexually active, with a husband/wife whom you believe to have been faithful to you. You also had a brief sexual affair about a year ago, but, as with your spouse, you use condoms as contraception, and have always done so. If asked about your sexual history, be vague and evasive.

Following these role plays, it is important to spend time in discussing not only the exchange in terms of the task set for the exercise, but also to consider the participants' feelings and experiences of being in the roles. This serves two purposes: to increase awareness on the part of the players of the emotional circumstances surrounding some of the health problems patients may experience. Second, because some of the role plays may prove to be emotionally threatening or demanding to participants from time to time, and talking about feelings derived from the role play exercise may help to minimize any residual disturbance left following the exercise.

This is especially the case in the following sections on dealing with emotions, breaking bad news, communicating with cancer patients and interactions with terminally ill or dying patients.

Discussion

1. Is it appropriate for health workers to pressure patients to reveal information they may not want to disclose? If so, under what circumstances might this be justified? What strategies might be used to minimize the problems in terms of disrupting the health worker–patient relationship?

2. What are the advantages and disadvantages of control during interview or health care interactions?

3. Is the negotiation of interview goals with the patient valuable in terms of health care? When should it not take place and why?

4. How much should patients be encouraged to participate in their own goal setting and how much responsibility should patients be encouraged to take for their own care?

5. Where patients opt out of decision making and responsibility for their own well being, under what circumstances is it legitimate for health workers to place the onus on the patients for their care?

8

Feelings: Your Own and Your Patient's

Educational Objectives

By the end of this chapter, you should be able to

- outline reasons for considering feelings in health care
- give reasons why feelings are often ignored during clinical communications
- list advantages and disadvantages to the staff of communications about feelings
- explain the importance of relating to the patient on an emotional level
- list three components of rapport
- differentiate between empathy and sympathy
- list means to establish empathy
- demonstrate the appropriate use of empathy and define empathic understanding
- give examples of verbal cues of emotional states
- give examples of non-verbal cues in emotional states
- recognize the importance of context in the interpretation of cues
- list appropriate responses to cues

Introduction

Feelings are probably the most ignored aspect of health related inter-actions. In almost every other area of life, feelings occupy a unique place determining to a large extent our behaviour (Frijda, 1986). Feelings are something we all have; they are part of our concrete experience of life; yet few, if any of us know much about them. We experience feelings without understanding them, and in some cases without recognizing what prompted them, which ones they were, or how they influenced us.

Feelings include emotions such as anger and joy as well as states like loneliness. Like the colours of the rainbow, feelings represent a spectrum of experience which can be divided up differently according to the language used to describe them. Our understanding of feelings is further complicated by the idiosyncratic meaning they may carry in addition to their sensory features. Also, there are clear cultural and sub-cultural differences in the labelling, recognition and expression of feelings (Ekman, 1972).

Communication of feeling is poorly understood. Darwin (1872) be-lieved the characteristic facial expressions accompanying different feeling states serve a communications role. More recently, research has identified some universal consistency in the interpretation of facial expression (Ekman, 1972). These universals are modified by culturally defined rules dictating the circumstances under which such expressions may be displayed (Ekman, 1972).

Biological models of emotions as primitive signalling devices both within and between individual members of our species receive a lot of attention, though they remain controversial (Harrè, Clarke and De Carlo, 1984). However, less attention has been paid to the social dimension of feelings. This is particularly true of models based of the social construc-tion of feelings (Averill, 1978). These propose a learned, symbolic signalling role for the expression of feelings (Lutz, 1988). Thus, interpretation of feeling is influenced by the context within which the expression occurs, and the past experience of the observer. These influences have been com-mented on elsewhere (Fielding and Tam, 1989).

Research emphasizes two different dimensions of feelings: the degree of arousal accompanying a feeling state, and the extent to which the feeling can be classified as positive or negative (pleasant or unpleasant).

Thought tends to precede feeling (Lazarus, 1984; Zajonc 1984). A sub-stantial body of research illustrates the change in feelings that can be achieved by the manipulation of thinking patterns (e.g. Ellis, 1958; Schacter, 1971; Beck, 1985). What is recognized is that the issues underpinning the relation-ship between cognitive activity (including thought, imagery, information processing and memory) and emotion are extremely complex (Williams, Watts, MacLeod and Mathews, 1988; Teasdale and Barnard, 1993).

How feeling states affect health is not clearly understood, yet since Hippocrates health practitioners have recognized the importance of the patient's feelings in determining well-being (Heberden, 1772). Recent research associates feelings with many areas of health. These include, but are not limited to, chronic diseases; acute diseases (Ramirez et al, 1989; Antoni and Goodkin, 1988; Fielding 1991); recovery from surgery (Egbert, et al, 1964; Janis, 1958; Ridgeway and Matthews, 1984); vulnerability to infectious diseases (Keicolt-Glaser 1987); duration of survival in cancer (Greer, Morris and Pettingale, 1978); onset of cardiac disease (Booth-Kewley and Friedman, 1987; Fielding 1991); neoplastic disease (Antoni and Goodkin, 1988); and autoimmune disorders (Solomon, 1981).

Thus feelings may have great biological importance in health care. Feelings are also important in human experience because they are significant in determining the quality of people's lives.

Why are feelings ignored in health care?

Why then are feelings so frequently overlooked or ignored by health workers? This can be largely attributed to two reasons. First, health workers' educational programmes fail to emphasize the importance of feelings. Second, many health workers are made very anxious by patients expressing their feelings.

Note how the failure of professional health worker training programmes to consider feelings — except as a specialty subject (e.g. psychology, psychiatry, psychiatric nursing and social work) — serves to reinforce the belief that feelings are not the concern of 'ordinary' nurses, doctors, and other health workers, when in fact they are.

Anxiety about patients' expression of feelings is rooted in several myths. First, some believe that if patients do express their feelings, this is in some way detrimental to patients and it reflects badly on the staff — 'What have you done? Why is the patient upset? Second, expressions of feeling tend to make health workers uneasy. Some health workers are anxious that allowing patients to express their emotion will open some kind of floodgate through which will pour a torrent of passions. When asked to follow this anticipated anxiety to its logical conclusion, most health workers see that this will only last for a short time, that it is largely harmless, and that violent emotion is exceptional.

Most health workers don't, however, follow this anxiety to its conclusion, and the result is that health workers end up fearing some horrible state where they would not be able to cope with the patient's feelings. Such anxieties may be at the root of the problem.

▨ Personal involvement: risks and benefits

Acknowledging and dealing with patients' feelings requires health workers to respond on a similar level. This may be very demanding emotionally. In some health care settings, such as paediatric oncology, the emotional demands on staff may lead to problems with occupational burnout. Under such circumstances, effective staff support is necessary if high staff turnover is to be avoided (see Chapter 13). However, the majority of health care is not so emotionally demanding and the need for emotional involvement will vary.

Crucially, by acknowledging and responding to patients' feelings, a health worker is responding to the patient as a *person*. Concern with the patient's feelings communicates concern for the patient's comfort — as a person, not simply a 'patient'. The quality of care patients perceive is likely to increase if the quality of communications is increased (Buller and Buller, 1988), and feelings are a fundamental component of communications.

The extent to which personal involvement should occur in health care settings is equivocal. It has been generally assumed that the health worker should 'handle' patients' feelings and emotions dispassionately, without any personal involvement. It is widely recommended that health workers do not burden their patients with biographic information about themselves. The reasons for this are as follows:

1. Patients who are having difficulties coping with aspects of their feelings may be made to feel more inadequate if they hear every one else can cope but they cannot.
2. Patients may feel pressured by the health worker which may make coping with their own feelings more difficult, violating the role prescriptions of doctors or nurses. If health workers are having difficulty coping, they should seek professional help, not discuss these problems with their patients.
3. A minority of patients may feel threatened for other reasons by the health worker's disclosure.
4. It risks generalizing the patients' experience, something which patients tend not to like.
5. It places an additional burden on patients when they are already under burden.

However, with care, the feelings of the health worker about exchanges with the patient can serve as a helpful tool to give feedback or to provide support to the patient.

Pt: How can I go back to work? Everyone will want to know why I

> got sick. People aren't stupid you know, they know about
> pneumonia in young people.

HW: It makes me feel angry to hear you talk like that. You sound like
you've given up already. Your family are going to feel the same
way. You fought hard to get well again. Don't give up now. You
can make it if you go back to work, I know it.

Through feedback from others, patients may come to realize that
their feelings are quite common and appropriate. That is, a patient's
feelings may be validated by a health worker sharing their own feelings
about the same or similar circumstances with the patients. This is in many
ways an extension to the empathic statement:

Pt: I just feel totally . . . oh, I don't know, fed up being in here.
HW: I can understand how that might feel, I get like that when I feel
unable to change things. It's hard.
Pt: If only there were something I could do about it!
HW: I don't know if it will help, but if I find myself in that kind of
situation, then by trying to distract myself from how helpless I
feel seems to make it easier to bear somehow.
Pt: Well, I suppose that makes sense. It's hard to distract yourself
in here: it's a constant reminder.

From the perspective of the health worker, the perception of involvement and, in exceptional circumstances, increasing vulnerability that arises
from more interaction on a feeling level requires a degree of openness and
self-confidence, which may take time to develop.

It can feel very threatening to a health worker to interact with a
patient on an emotional level. There is a fine balance to be maintained
between being too involved and being too professionally distant. The
optimum involves dealing with emotional issues as needed, while maintaining a level of professionalism. The health worker cannot be a friend to
each patient, but may at times be a confidant.

There are no rules for how much involvement is best. The advantages
of involvement are that greater empathy, closeness and support can be
achieved and this improves quality of care. The disadvantages are that too
much involvement can begin to interfere with care, affect judgement and
be emotionally damaging for both patient and health worker. By contrast,
little or no involvement gives the impression of being cold, distant and
uncaring.

Greater attention needs to be paid to patients' feeling states and from
time to time this may make emotional demands on the health worker.
While closeness to people is generally considered desirable, there are times

when it is inadvisable to get close emotionally with certain patients. The patient may hook in to some aspect of the health worker's needs or sensitivities, which can handicap the health worker when it comes to objective decision making about the patient.

A difficult problem arises when the health worker or the patient experiences romantic or sexual feelings towards the other. For ethical reasons, health workers are discouraged from this, and doctors are prohibited. Most staff keep their feelings to themselves if they do develop affections for patients. There are unfortunately frequent occurrences where patients, usually male patients, make sexual or romantic advances to female health workers. It is important that health workers be assertive and confident in dealing with these situations. The patient who makes derogatory, sexist or sexual comments to a nurse can be best dealt with by ignoring any comment of this type and not responding to the patient when he speaks in this way. However, acceptable speech should be responded to quite normally. This seems to be the way many nurses deal with such situations.

Different strategies may need to be adopted in order to help colleagues cope better with these and other stressful effects on the unit staff. (See Chapter 13.)

Relating to the patient

The relationship between the health worker and the patient is very important at all times, but especially so where the discussion of emotions are concerned. Sharing feelings with another person may be more difficult than giving clinical details about a disease. A health worker who is unable to relate well emotionally may experience difficulty in understanding and empathizing with patients who wish to discuss their feelings.

Two main processes, rapport and empathy, are fundamentally involved in relating to others.

Rapport

Rapport is important for all communication. It is particularly important that health workers who will be dealing with emotional elements of patients' problems be able to develop a sense of rapport with their patients. Rapport has been defined as

> . . . a relationship based on a high degree of community of thought, interest and sentiment (Drever, 1969).

Stewart (1983) emphasizes three important components of rapport: harmony, compatibility and affinity. Rapport is being on the same wavelength, or in tune, with a person. Rapport constitutes the foundation of effective therapeutic relationships, without which health workers and patients will not hear each other. They therefore do not communicate effectively. This makes helping with emotional aspects of patients' problems unlikely.

If rapport is not established, blaming the patient, self, or others is not helpful. Rapport requires two people's participation. Either may find the other incompatible and be unable to establish a fruitful therapeutic relationship. Avoid biasing colleagues against the patient with labels like 'a problem patient', 'awkward' or 'difficult'. These commonly used terms are unhelpful. Blaming is unproductive. The patient may be responsible but blame will not rectify the situation. There may be important reasons (to the patient) why this occurs. These need to be explored and understood.

Rapport is important in all relationships if they are to be effective for communication. So though we are discussing rapport in the section on emotions, it is relevant to all levels of communication.

Trust is an important element in rapport. If a health worker is untrustworthy, patients or colleagues are unlikely to be willing to share with that health worker. This is particularly so when dealing with children, who, once trust is lost, are exceedingly unwilling to reinstate it.

Empathy

Empathy refers to the ability to enter into an appreciation of another's thoughts, feelings or experiences. Definitions vary; for instance, the concise Oxford Dictionary defines it as 'the power of identifying oneself mentally with a person or object of contemplation', whereas Chambers 20th Century defines it as 'the experiencing of another's feelings, etc., by the power of imagination'. One of my students once defined it as 'the insertion of one person into another'. All these definitions give the flavour of imagining another's experiences in a parallel fashion to your own. This requires the health workers to take on the perspective of the patients, considering their perceptions of a situation, and inducing within themselves the likely experiences that derive from such perspectives. In essence, it is stepping into the patients' world and sharing it with them, or inserting yourself into another's life and experiencing the world from another's point of view.

Empathy, not sympathy

Empathy is not absolute, but graded; it varies from time to time, with patient to patient, or staff to staff. It can be gained, increased, decreased and lost. It is not sympathy, though sympathy requires empathic appreciation of another's circumstance. Sympathy is feeling *for* that person. Empathy is feeling *with* that person.

This is an important distinction. It is important because sympathy seldom helps the person who is suffering but empathy can be very helpful indeed.

Empathy is important for dealing with emotional aspects of health and illness. Appreciation of the anxiety or fear caused by a forthcoming operation, or a 'suspicious lump' will go a long way towards understanding the emotional needs of the patient. This in turn can make the identification of effective coping strategies for the patient much easier.

HW:	How do you feel today?
Pt:	Oh, much the same, you know.
HW:	Down?
Pt:	Yeah. The back's really uncomfortable. I just can't get comfortable.
HW:	It must be be hard to cope with. (empathic statement)
Pt:	I don't know. I, I don't . . . want to have to go through this every day.
HW:	Yes. I imagine it would make you feel pretty depressed. (empathic statement)
Pt:	It . . . does. I don't see, ah, any future . . . I, . . . (becomes tearful)
HW:	(stays silent and involved)
Pt:	(sigh!)
HW:	Is it difficult to see a way out?
Pt:	(nods)

The health worker makes a guess that the patient is not feeling good, based on the patient's initial response. This requires empathy. The patient is experiencing an understandable reaction to a chronic pain problem which needs to be addressed if it is not to cause problems for the patient in future. To understand this is to begin to see what life might be like from the patient's perspective. The empathic response of the health worker enables both parties to share the difficulties experienced by the patient and this may lead to consideration of how best to cope with the problems, both physical and emotional. Not only does empathy help the patient, it can also help the health worker better appreciate the patient's experience. This can significantly improve quality of care.

> ## Key Points
>
> Establish empathy by:
> * sharing feelings with the person
> * use of empathic statements
> * 'hearing' what the person is saying
> * trying to adopt the others' perspective
>
> Try to understand the other person's view by imagining self in the others' situation, discussing how it might feel.

Feeling cues

Most health workers have as much intuitive knowledge about emotional cues as the next person. Much of our socialization as children is taken up in learning to interpret the social signals of other people, though there are those whose social skills are poor, or who are more inward focused in their perceptions and less sensitive to the behaviour of others. There are many levels of indicators about the feeling state of others, be they patients, staff, or colleagues. Some of these have already been outlined in Chapter 5. For convenience of discussion, these can be divided into verbal and non-verbal indicators. Though the two are usually present together, they can and do occur individually. These cues can be responded to in different ways.

Responding

Failure to respond to cues

A person can fail to detect or recognize a cue as indicating feeling states. Some health workers have this difficulty, but it is the exception rather than the rule. A more common pattern is recognition of emotional cues followed by some strategy for avoidance, such as a redirection of the attention away from the cue or topic, or pretending not to notice a cue.

Pt: How long am I likely to be in hospital?

HW: Not too long. If everything goes all right you'll be home after a week.

Pt: Everything's going to be all right, isn't it?

HW: Has the technician come to get a blood sample today?

A common alternative is for the cue to be recognized, but instead of dealing directly with the issue, the health worker offers what is generally called 'reassurance'. However, reassurance is all too often used to avoid dealing with emotional material, hence it fails to be true reassurance.

Pt: How long am I likely to be in hospital?
HW: Not too long. If everything goes all right you'll be home after a week.
Pt: Everything's going to be all right, isn't it?
HW: Of course. Now don't you worry. Has the technician come to get a blood sample today?

Failure to respond doesn't necessarily indicate intent to avoid. The health worker may simply fail to recognize that a statement is a cue, as may be the case in the first example. Provision of reassurance is more often seen as being all that is necessary to satisfy the patient's requirements.

In each case above, the response of the health worker shuts off any discussion of the topic or discourages further discussion by reassuring. The most beneficial approach is to invite further discussion.

Responding to cues

Responding to a cue requires first acknowledgement, followed by clarification.

Pt: How long am I likely to be in hospital?
HW: Not too long. If everything goes all right you'll be home after a week.
Pt: Everything's going to be all right, isn't it?
HW: Are you worried about the operation?

While this picks up the cue, it *assumes* a cause for the patient's concern, which may be more or less obvious, but may also be incorrect. Another way to pick up the cue offered by the patient, which avoids such assumptions, is to use a reflective form of response.

Pt: How long am I likely to be in hospital?
HW: Not too long. If everything goes all right you'll be home after a week.
Pt: Everything's going to be all right, isn't it?
HW: What makes you ask that?
or,
Pt: How long am I likely to be in hospital?

HW: Not too long. If everything goes all right you'll be home after a week.

Pt: Everything's going to be all right, isn't it?

HW: Going to be all right . . . . ?

The use of reflection here is most appropriate, giving the patient room to respond and express concerns and for the health worker to obtain more information about these concerns before deciding how to respond. The response might simply be reassurance, or information or more detailed discussion of the patient's problems.

The kinds of responses health workers might make to emotional cues depend on the individual style of the health worker, but here are some responses that may be appropriate to make:

> You don't seem very happy today.
> I hear you had some bad news, would you like to talk about it?
> There's a very worried look on your face. Is something troubling you?

Most people already have a good selection of responses suitable for such occasions. Sometimes, a non-verbal response may be more appropriate, such as taking hold of a patient's hand, or just taking a moment to sit next to a patient in silence. The patient may not want to discuss the problem at the particular moment.

By emphasizing these points, educating health workers on the importance of responding to cues, and by reassuring (and perhaps even holding a discussion on health workers' feelings about patients' emotions), the use of lack of understanding as an excuse will be reduced significantly. Anxiety about patients' feelings may also be significantly reduced. Often health workers need only be told that it is quite acceptable to allow patients to express feelings, that it is not harmful, and is often helpful to the patients, for the health worker to be more prepared to deal with emotions. Health workers who still discourage or avoid dealing with emotional cues may need more individual assistance or even counselling.

Cues among younger children

Children's behaviour is often the most obvious cue to how they are feeling. Younger children are inclined to be happy and to play when they feel secure. When they do not feel this way they seldom appear happy and, though they may still play, the nature of their play is increasingly coloured by their internal experiences. Hence, children who are angry may be particularly aggressive with their toys — dolls and cars may be smacked, shouted at or crashed for being 'bad'. 'Badness' is a key dimension for many young children as they are quick to perceive moral judgement in the actions of others towards them, and vice versa. Fear or anxiety is the other major dimension of childhood feeling that will be commonly seen in health care settings. The anxious child clings to its caretaker, unhappy to be left alone even for a moment. The fear may be externalized onto imaginary aspects of the child's environment, such as 'monsters'.

Children aged between six months and four years are particularly vulnerable to separation from the main caretaker and can become severely withdrawn if hospitalized without an accompanying caretaker. This withdrawal occurs only after an initial stage of extreme protestation, crying, refusal to eat and unwillingness to be comforted by others. The withdrawal phase is often interpreted by staff as settling down, but this is not the case. Children in the withdrawal phase are essentially in a state of bereavement; though they may appear to be superficially interacting or cooperative, they are usually quite depressed.

Verbal cues

False reassurance

The nature of verbal cues varies. Some verbal cues will be more apparent than others, especially those that are intentional cues, whereas unintentional cues will be less obvious. A statement such as 'I'm very worried', or 'I'm frightened' appears clear and unambiguous, but may still be responded to with 'reassurance'. Of course, phrases like 'everything will be all right', or 'don't worry' slip easily off the tongue, but these really only serve to discourage communication. In offering prompt reassurance, the implicit message to the patient is that the health worker is not willing to discuss the matter. The patient usually accedes to this. There are certainly many cases where providing 'reassurance' is unconsciously intended to serve just such a purpose.

Less obvious are the verbal cues that appear among other material, which the observant health workers can pick out to present back to the patient to gain clarification.

Pt: . . . It wouldn't be so bad me being sick all the time if my son wasn't so demanding. Do you know how long I'll be in here?

HW: You should be out in a few days. You said your son was demanding. Does he make life difficult for you?

Pt: Oh, he never stops. He's always after something.

HW: Don't the rest of your family help?

In this example, the health worker picks up the cue about the patient's son and uses that to expand enquiry into the patient's family background, which may be aggravating the patient's complaint, or interfering with the patient's ability to cope. This should not be overlooked where there is no obvious cause for a problem. Many apparent cues may fail to be other than off-the-cuff statements by a patient. It is fairly easy to tune into individual patients' styles of disclosure of information, especially if you spend time to get to know patients a little as people, and this makes picking out the cues a lot easier.

Non-verbal cues

Rarely do verbal cues occur without non-verbal cues. The opposite is much more likely to be the case, with non-verbal cues occurring in the absence of verbal cues.

A group of behaviours which might be thought of as non-verbal vocal behaviour, or para-linguistic utterances as they have been called by speech investigators, includes the following:
* uhms and ahs
* pauses in speech
* change of tone or texture of voice
* stuttering or stammering in otherwise unaffected speech
* sighing

These kinds of speech behaviours are ambiguous on their own. However, they can serve as cues, especially in the presence of other non-verbal indicators, such as the following:
* direction of gaze
* change in eye-contact
* change in posture or stiffening of posture
* change or stiffening of facial expression
* increased restlessness or fidgeting
* picking at nails
* tears or moistening of the eyes
* chewing or biting of the lip or fingernails
* rubbing together of hands or hands rubbing on legs
* crossing or re-crossing of the legs
* tapping or flicking of the foot
* blushing
* (combinations of the above)
* hostility

These non-verbal cues may indicate, with varying degrees of certainty, emotionally sensitive elements of the interview. Together with verbal cues, they give the strongest indication of the person being affected.

Key Points

Non-verbal cues may indicate discomfort or emotional arousal. However, the meaning of these cues has to be interpreted in the context of the discussion. Talking about certain topics may cause this reaction, not because it is a problem for the patient, but because the patient is not used to discussing such topics — marital relations, sexuality, etc. — with a stranger.

People may display these individual behaviours, but most often non-verbal cues will occur in certain combinations that we are mostly familiar with. One person may look 'worried', another may look 'depressed', a third 'upset' or 'distressed', and a fourth may be angry, aggressive and uncooperative, and so on. These are social interpretations of feeling states; as a result they are more familiar to us as emotional or mood states and provide another level of cue about how the interviewee may be feeling. This brings us close to empathy once more.

Aggression or anger in patients is something that many health workers have difficulty responding to. Defensiveness in the health worker indicates a perception that the patient's aggressiveness is a personal attack, rather than as a means of self-defense for the patient. It is important to remember that hostility often indicates a frightened patient. This patient needs understanding, not response in kind, though firm responses may be warranted at times.

Stan was 37 years old, married with two young children, and was awaiting insurance payment for a foot injury sustained in his work as a security guard. He suffered a small inferior myocardial infarction, and during hospitalization was uncooperative, continuing to smoke cigarettes and repeatedly threatening to discharge himself. He eventually left hospital against advice and was readmitted two months later with an extension of the initial infarct. Again he was uncooperative and discharged himself, only to be readmitted two or three days later with chest pain. He was eventually given haloperidol, chlorpromazine and diazepam in order to 'stop him removing his drips' and to make him less fractious. He was never violent but he appeared intimidating. He still insisted on smoking against advice. He underwent angiography (the result of which was ambiguous) and, nonetheless, angioplasty, was discharged, readmitted one week later with chest pain, but no reinfarction. He required six hourly pethidine to control his chest pain. Repeat angiography showed all coronary arteries remained clear.

The Coronary Care Unit staff, both doctors and nurses, responded to Stan as a problem patient. In spite of a medical and nursing diagnosis of 'anxious', he was treated as though he were behaving badly on purpose. Staff were at a loss as to how to deal with his desire to discharge himself. The staff perceived his situation as life-threatening and thought it obvious that he would want to stay in hospital, where he could be treated. The staff failed to understand why he would repeatedly discharge himself and continue to smoke. Eventually, it was realized that Stan was very frightened about dying, had financial problems at home, and was extremely afraid of hospitals. (His mother had been misdiagnosed, therefore wrongly treated, and died as a result in the same hospital.) Though his behaviour was powered by the anxiety the staff recognized early on, his rather inadequate coping meant that he could not or did not use the kinds of cognitive or similar avoidance skills many patients in a similar situation would have used. The result was frustration and anger.

Stan was also frustrated by the fact that he wanted to view himself as healthy, but was affected by a chronic condition. His frustration was directed at the staff who were unable to 'cure' him. He thus felt trapped and blamed the staff (they being, apparently, the most obvious and accessible) to whom he directed his aggression.

The failure of the staff to appreciate that inadequate coping skills may motivate aggressive and uncooperative behaviour led to the 'us against him' perception. The staff therefore gave up attempts to understand his behaviour. The label 'problem patient' generated more difficulty, consigning the patient to a category which needed to be overcome before a more therapeutic relationship could be established. The patient didn't trust the hospital and feared for his life, preferring to risk his chances more with his family than with the hospital, but needed hospital expertise to deal with his unstable chest pain (much of it related to emotional factors), while feeling frustrated that the health workers didn't cure his symptoms.

This example illustrates how staff and patient can become alienated, leading to considerable difficulties, greater loss of efficiency and loss of unit morale and how aggressiveness, frustration and anxiety are often intermingled.

Stan was a difficult patient to manage. But he wasn't a problem patient. However, there were problems in his management. The staff failed to recognize the contribution to his problem brought on by Stan's circumstances; threatened, dependent, lacking control (even over whether he could smoke!). Instead, his behaviour was seen to reflect his personality. This is called Fundamental Attribution Error, the belief that these behaviours reflect traits of the person, rather than being a result of the person's circumstances.

His situation was made easier by several approaches. Increasing the amount of control Stan had over his behaviour was a first step. (Allowing him to smoke was probably less harmful cardiologically than the constant pressure of frustration he experienced when smoking was prohibited.) Giving him permission to be mobile at will, even negotiating G.T.N. and pethedine dosage (within limits) was eventually agreed to by the consultant in charge. This was done after careful explanation to Stan that he was in a bind. By smoking and not resting, he was increasing his cardiac risk, but that he could choose which he wanted. He chose to walk off the ward and smoke outside (much to the horror of the staff, to whom this was attempted suicide!). He obtained more control over his situation.

By using a more empathic approach, acknowledging the patient's feelings and helping the patient to understand these himself, both staff and patient could have been spared a lot of tension and anger over the situation.

Concurrently, he was seen by a clinical psychologist attached to the Coronary Care Unit who worked to help Stan develop more appropriate coping skills. Stan eventually recovered from his acute admission, though his stay was undoubtedly extended by a mixture of his anxiety and smoking. He remained hostile, however, whenever he was required to attend follow-up appointments. He has stopped smoking, exercises regularly and has lost weight, but he continues to find hospitals difficult!

Eliciting feelings

The techniques of eliciting patients' feelings have been discussed in Chapter 6. A brief summary of previously mentioned techniques for eliciting feelings involves:
- asking about current feelings
- asking about past feelings
- asking patient to recall a situation that evoked a similar feeling
- asking patient to describe the parts of their body affected by feelings
- using metaphor and simile to describe feelings

Use of direct questions about feelings will, in most instances, open discussion:

> How did that make you feel?
> What were you feeling then?
> Did that feel bad?
> Are you feeling upset?

Some patients tend to give a response based on what they thought. Return to feelings by saying something like:

HW: That's what you thought, but how did it feel?
Pt: How did it feel? Oh, well, . . .

Empathic questions help in relating to the patient and encouraging the exploration of the emotional side of the patient's problem:

> I think I would be scared of my first operation.
> You don't seem your usual self today. That makes me feel there's something bothering you.
> I guess things look pretty bleak from your viewpoint?

Generally, relating to patients', or colleagues' feelings and emotions requires the health worker to show personal feelings. Self-awareness is important. Some health workers see dealing with emotions and feelings as daunting, but if the patient or staff are treated with respect and unconditional positive regard, and the health worker is non-judgemental and warm, much of the difficulty goes out of such interactions.

Summary

- Don't be afraid of patients' feelings and emotions: relating to feelings makes the patient feel that you are relating to them as a person, not simply a medical or nursing case.
- Effective relationships need a basic orientation of the health workers. This should include:
    - respect for the person
    - unconditional positive regard
    - non-judgmental attitude
    - warm manner
- Rapport is crucial to effective discussion of feelings and forms the foundation, or carrier wave on which good communication is based.

- Empathic understanding, appreciation of the person's experience by the health workers 'putting themselves in the others' shoes'
- Establish empathy by:
  - sharing feelings with the person
  - use of empathic statements
  - 'hearing' what the person is saying
  - trying to adopt the others' perspective
- The meaning of emotional behaviours, as with all other behaviour, must be considered in the context of the circumstances of the person.
- Aggressiveness is often a defense against anxiety or fear.
- Avoid using labels like 'problem patient'.
- Be aware of and respond to emotional cues.

Exercises

Some of these exercises might be upsetting for some students as they deal with emotionally difficult situations. After the exercises are completed, allow at least 15 to 30 minutes for the students to discuss their feelings about the role plays and their own roles therein. This is itself a useful exercise in both self-awareness and in empathic development.

1. *You are the health worker.* Your patient has recently been admitted to your general surgery ward for exploratory surgery following sustained weight loss. Medical examination has proved to be negative, though some biochemical indicators (serum alkaline phosphatase in particular) are raised. Your first visit to this patient after coming on duty suggests that he or she may be anxious. Your task is to identify the main reasons for the patient's anxiety. You have seven minutes.

    You are the patient. You have been losing weight steadily over the last two months and your appetite is poor. Your doctor has not been able to find a reason for your weight loss. He has sent you into hospital for a medical workout, and the physicians have transferred you to this ward. They said something about surgery, but you did not fully understand. Be yourself as much as possible, but consider the possibility that there may be something seriously wrong.

2. *You are the health worker.*   For two days, you have been caring for a patient who is known to be HIV positive. The patient is currently being treated for a sudden pneumonia and is making good recovery. The patient stops you and asks if you have time to talk.

    You are the patient.   You know that you are a carrier of HIV but have been trying particularly hard to use every positive thinking, good diet approach you can find to help yourself to recover. Two days ago, you developed a fever and were brought into hospital with a diagnosis of pneumonia. This has responded well to antibiotics and you feel much better today. You are worried about the future. You do not know what to do to help yourself. You are scared. Be yourself as much as possible. You have asked to talk with the nurse who has been caring for you. You want to know what is likely to happen in future regarding your health.

3. *You are the relative.*   Your five-year-old daughter/sister has been treated for leukemia two years ago and is not showing any signs of recurrence. However, as a consequence of the treatment she received, she has increasingly shown signs of difficulty in coping with school and shows poor speech development. You have asked to see a practitioner to discuss her problem. You are very upset about the effect that the treatment has had and feel it bitterly unfair that having had leukemia she now has other problems to deal with. Be yourself as much as possible.

    You are the health worker.   The relative asking to see you has a five-and-a-half year old daughter successfully treated for acute lymphoblastic leukemia two-and-a-half years ago. However, there has been some neurological complication from the treatment administered at the time. This is known to have been moderately severe and the child is now mildly intellectually handicapped.

Discussion

1. When patients are upset or show signs of emotional disturbance, but do not seek help, should staff encourage them to discuss their feelings, or should privacy be respected?

2. Under what circumstances would you consider it inappropriate for a patient to initiate discussion of their feelings with a health worker, and why?

3. Should staff discuss their own feelings and life experiences with their patients, if they think this will help the patient? If no, why not? If yes, under what circumstances?

4. Do you think staff groups are a good idea? Would you encourage one on your unit, or do you think they are unnecessary? If so, why?

9

Exposition: Giving Information to Patients

Educational Objectives

By the end of this chapter, you should be able to

- list the main reasons for non-adherence with treatment
- list the main reasons why physicians and other health workers fail to provide appropriate levels of information to patients
- recognize the role of medical jargon in patient misunderstanding and confusion
- recognize the value in organizing information before this is given to the patient
- recognize the advantages of giving precise information rather than general information
- recognize the importance of considering the patient's belief system (world view) before information giving
- recognize the need for non-jargon terminology when giving information to a patient
- recognize the influence of information sequence on subsequent recall
- recognize the role of emphasis and repetition
- list the components of explicit categorization
- recognize the importance of explicit categorization for improving patient recall of information
- recognize the improved recall associated with combining different techniques for recall

▨ **Introduction**

Chapters 9 to 11 focus on information giving or exposition. Chapter 9 outlines two main areas of information giving, techniques for assessing information need and for giving information to maximize recall. Chapter 10 considers the special problems of handling difficult questions from patients. Chapter 11 focuses on disclosing bad news to the patient.

Ley and Spelman (1972) first reported the relationship between exposition and subsequent adherence to treatment. The importance of patients following treatment recommendations is self-evident. Yet, if patients either do not understand or forget the instructions given to them, then they cannot adhere to treatment goals. These reasons remain major causes of non-adherence to treatment (Ley, 1984).

Conversely, by depriving patients of information, two things happen. First, they are unable to predict the nature, extent or timing of demands that the illness will make on them, or plan how best to cope with these demands. Because they cannot predict the timing and extent of demand, uncertainty and stress is much more likely. Second, the patients are forced into a passive role as a recipient of health care and stay this way while health care staff control information. The patients are more likely to feel helpless and dependent on health professionals (Thorne, 1993). This is the opposite of what should be happening. Effective health care means teaching self-reliance and responsibility in health maintenance and care.

Increasing patient understanding involves informing the patient in a manner the patient is likely to understand. In Chapter 2 we identified the association between memory encoding and recall. By definition, understanding is the grasping of meaning. Therefore, increasing the meaningfulness of information for the patient should improve its recall.

The active nature of memory is influenced by many factors that can affect later recall of information. Important among these factors are the following: environmental distractions; level of attention; the nature of the material to be memorized; the simultaneous or subsequent presentation of similar or related information; how the material is presented; the memory strategies used by the learner; the emotional state of the learner at the time of presentation and recall; and the presence or absence of cues at the time of recall.

By the use of simple preparation and basic techniques, many of these problems can be easily overcome. This can increase substantially patient understanding of the information given by the health worker. This in turn helps maximize the likelihood that instructions will be adhered to. It can also increase patient satisfaction with communications. Overall, this may result in significant improvements in patient adherence with recommended treatment.

Problems with information giving

Poor information giving is perhaps the most common reason for patient dissatisfaction. The problems in information giving can be classified into practitioner- or manager-related and patient- or staff-related problems.

Practitioner-related problems

An important first step to effective information giving is to use an approach to care that does not fragment responsibility for the patient. So, one doctor (or nurse) needs to take overall responsibility for the patient, no matter how many other doctors become involved. In nursing care, patient-oriented care rather than task-oriented care can help avoid diffusion of responsibility. In other health professions, individualized care programmes may only be possible in so far as there are more than one or two staff members on a unit at any one time. Multidisciplinary team care is increasingly widespread, yet often fails to adopt a policy decision about information management. This significantly increases the risk of fragmented information care.

Few patients receive as much information as they desire about their health and care. Studies show that most patients want as much information about their condition as possible, even when the news might be considered 'bad' (Blanchard et al, 1988). When health workers are asked why they don't give information to patients, a number of reasons are given. These include:
- a belief that patients don't want information
- a belief that someone else has given the patients all the information they desire
- a lack of time
- a belief that patients don't need to know information
- a belief that information may in some way be harmful or interfere with patient management
- a belief that giving information to the patient will damage the patient's cooperativeness

Exploring these beliefs one at a time is revealing. Most of these reasons do not stand up to close scrutiny.

Patients don't want information

Most patients want information on all aspects of their condition. It makes no difference if the information is good news or bad. Information reduces uncertainty, and uncertainty is stressful. For most people, the uncertainty of not knowing what is happening is more difficult to bear than the certainty of bad news. Some patients do not want bad news, but these are in the minority; these patients will, if asked, express their unwillingness to be kept informed.

Someone else has given the patient information

The style of care that is used fundamentally affects the priorities given to the psychosocial needs of the patient. Where there is no policy about information giving, the belief that someone else has given the information to the patient is often widespread. The result is often that no one tells the patient.

To avoid this, the patient's level of knowledge, understanding and information about his or her circumstances must be assessed. In so doing, any gaps in information will become apparent, and these can be met. Thus, despite what someone else may or may not have told the patient, it is important for the health worker to evaluate the patient's knowledge. There remains the need for the health worker to provide updates and specialist health advice. Also the role as an information resource is on-going. There is no excuse for failing to check the patient's need for information.

Lack of time to give information

Lack of time is the most common excuse for not informing patients. It is unacceptable. To dismiss information giving due to a shortage of time is also false economy. By not providing information, patient satisfaction is reduced, and patients are less likely to adhere to treatment. As such they are more likely to make further or repeated use of health services. In this way, patients contribute more to the workload, and thus to the shortage of time. By giving more and better information, patient satisfaction is higher, with the result that treatment is adhered to and therefore more likely to be effective, thus achieving better use of scarce resources.

There is a second argument against shortage of time. The importance of information is such that it warrants a higher priority in the care hierarchy. If time is insufficient, then decisions will need to be made about the priorities for care. Administrative tasks, though important, should not take precedence over care. The only purpose of administration is to enable service. Administration should not be an end in itself. By delegating administrative duties to non-clinical staff, more time can be released for care by clinical staff.

Patients don't need to know

Beliefs that patients don't need to know information about their condition produce very dissatisfied patients. Irrespective of what patients may or may not need to know, the evidence is incontrovertible that the vast majority of people *want* to know as much as they can about their illness, diagnosis, and perhaps to a lesser extent, prognosis (Blanchard et al, 1988).

It is also a moot point about what patients need to know. Who is so knowledgeable as to say what people do or don't need to know to live their lives? The patients are the best judges of what they think they need to know. To deny patients information about themselves when they want such information reflects a lack of respect for the patients.

Patients may be harmed by information

A similar case holds for the mistaken belief that information may be in some way harmful to the patient. Information alone is not harmful. Even when the prognosis suggests death, in the majority of instances the patient still wants to know (Cartwright, 1964; Ley and Spelman, 1967; Blanchard et al, 1988). The arguments against information harming patients are detailed in Chapter 11.

Information giving may interfere with management

The argument that giving information to patients will interfere with their management is debatable. There is a growing ethical requirement that the informed consent presently required for procedures should extend to informed participation in decision making. These arguments are also explored in detail in Chapter 11.

So we can see that none of the arguments used to justify the position of not giving information to patients stand up to challenge, and can only be upheld by a continuing adherence to an outmoded philosophy of health care. As has happened in the USA, consumer pressure will eventually force a change of practice in many other countries not yet providing the level of information giving that patients desire.

Children are just as capable of understanding information if given at an appropriate level. There are no reasons why children should not also be given information. There may be an even stronger case for keeping children informed. Because children can't vote doesn't mean they can feel insecure, helpless and stressed. They also have fewer coping resources at their disposal than adults, so they need to have available resources — like information — maximized.

The problem doesn't stop at failure to give information. Studies where practitioners felt they had made specific attempts to give patients information have still resulted in high levels of patient dissatisfaction with communications (Spelman et al, 1966; Houghton, 1968). So even when practitioners make extra effort to give information, patients may not get the message.

Patient-related problems

What about the problems that can be ascribed to the patient? These have been less well documented, but may be as important as practitioner-related problems and no less amenable to change. Patients may be given information repeatedly, only to say later that they were told nothing by anyone.

As part of a study on recovery from acute myocardial infarction, patients' information recall was explored. During hospitalization patients were informed at least three times regarding diagnosis and recovery progress. Following discharge patients had two out-patient appointments (during which further information on recovery was given), and also attended a six-hour rehabilitation programme running over 12 weeks following discharge (which was specifically aimed at educational goals). They were given a booklet containing information about recovery from heart attacks. Six months later patients were asked to recall what they had been told about their illness during their hospital stay. Eighty percent of patients questioned said they had been told nothing at any time about their illness (Fielding, 1984).

In this study, patients had been given a large volume of information in both spoken and written form. However, few failed to recollect anything they were told (or at least admit to recollecting anything). When questioned, most of the patients admitted reading the information booklet in a cursory manner when first given it, then putting it in a drawer on returning home and forgetting about it. In many cases, patients felt that the information contained in the booklet was not the kind of information they wanted. The rehabilitation programme apparently failed to increase information recall for patients. Yet this was a major aim of the exercise. Such findings are particularly worrying when health workers make specific efforts to increase information giving and efforts fail.

This and other studies serve to illustrate the importance of using correct exposition techniques and of providing information patients want.

Clearly, there are times when patients do not pay attention to what is being said, where misunderstandings occur and are not clarified. Although patient problems exist, it is principally the health worker's responsibility to maximize the accessibility, comprehensibility and retention of information given to patients.

Preparation for information giving

During this and the subsequent two chapters, we will be developing a model of information giving called ADA. ADA has three components, hence its name:

Assessment
Disclosure
Assimilation

In this chapter, we will explore the first of the ADA components, assessment of information needs.

Preliminary needs assessment

Assessment of information needs must be carried out on two levels. First, on initial contact or admission of patients, they must be asked clearly whether or not they want to be kept informed of their circumstances. The health worker is then aware of the patient's desire for information and involvement during investigations and treatment.

Second, prior to information giving, a more detailed assessment of the patient's need for information should be made. The health worker then knows how much and what kind of information is needed.

Admission assessment

On first contact with a patient, an assessment of the extent of the patient's desire for information and involvement needs to be made. This should be done on first contact when other information is gathered for two reasons. First, the collection of this information becomes incorporated in planning and implementing the patient's care. Second, if these questions are asked later they tend to strongly indicate bad news is imminent. Imagine asking a patient after tests for weight loss, 'If we were to have found anything bad, like cancer, would you want us to tell you about it?' This is clearly an inappropriate way to disclose bad news. During initial contact assessment the question is unobtrusive and this makes it the optimal time to gather such information.

Angell (1984) recommends three questions to be asked of the patient, to avoid health workers (particularly physicians and nurses) misunderstanding a patient's wishes about informing family members:

1. Do you wish to be fully informed of medical findings and consulted on all important decisions during your hospitalization?
2. If so, do you have any objections to having your family informed as well as yourself?
3. If you do not wish to fully informed, would you like to designate a family member or someone else to be kept informed instead?

In asking these questions, the health worker identifies the extent to which the patient wishes to be kept informed. These questions are best asked as part of an admission interview.

Specific assessment of needs

Before prescribing medication or nursing interventions for a patient, an assessment is always carried out of the patient's need for treatment. This involves identifying what the problem is, and then identifying the appropriate intervention. Before giving information, it is important to follow a similar procedure first. This avoids the potential problems of:

1. giving insufficient information
2. giving too much information
3. giving the wrong kind of information

Therefore, an information assessment is carried out. This is simply done and requires identifying what the patient's information needs currently are.

The main steps to information assessment are as follows:

1. Identify patients' understanding of their problem.
2. Identify patients' current concerns about their situation.
3. Ask the patients if they need or want any information in addition to that they have already been given.

1. Identify patients' understanding of their problem.   This is important. Remember, patients may have a very different conception of their problem to the health worker.

It is widely assumed that patients will accept unquestionably any information offered to them. Yet there are good grounds to question whether this is the case. Consider the following example.

You complain of repeated laryngitis and upper respiratory tract infections. You consult a practitioner. He tells you that your complaint is due to a disturbance in the flow of energy throughout your body. This causes high levels of energy to build up in some parts, while other parts have much less energy than they need. Consequently, certain faulty 'components' in your body need to be 'adjusted' so that a blockage in the circuits of your body can be relieved. Treatment involves having small piles of smoldering herbs held close to your skin over different parts of your body.

Presented with this explanation for an illness, how many of us would agree to having small fires ignited on different parts of our body as a remedy? This conceptualization clashes quite strongly with common allopathic, Western concepts of illness causality and treatment. It is likely that this explanation and treatment would be seen by the majority as lacking credibility, with consequent non-adherence to the treatment.

Yet, isn't this what we expect of some of our patients? Many patients have world views that differ from those of allopathic medicine. A biochemical or bacterial explanation of disease may seem as strange and incredible to them. That such patients don't take the antibiotics as prescribed is hardly surprising. As for the energy model of disease and its associated treatment, a similar one is widely recognized and continues to be used to good effect in China.

Therefore, it can be very useful before offering explanations to patients to consider the their own concepts of health and disease. Asking the patient,

What do you think is the problem?

may help to find out. Of course the patient may reply,

You tell me! That's why I've come here.

However, almost all patients already have some ideas about their problem before they consult a practitioner (Nerenz and Leventhal, 1983). They will also have some causal attributions about the factors precipitating their complaint. They will be all too willing to reveal these if asked. An understanding of these factors indicates the kind of world model patients may hold. It can also indicate patients' perception of their own ability to control or modify these perceived causes. Where the perceived causes are improbable, it may indicate the need for an educationally focused discussion directed at modifying patients' understanding.

Don't be afraid to explore patients' understanding of their condition particularly if it differs from the allopathic model.

> ### Key point:
>
> Find out
> - what the patient believes is the problem
> - what the patient believes is causing the problem
> - what the patient thinks should be done about it

2. Identify patients' current concerns about their situation.   In addition to patients' understanding of the problem, the health worker should attempt to identify the patient's current concerns. That is, what, if anything, is worrying the patient at present. This can be achieved by the following style of question:

Is your problem very much of a worry for you?

followed by,

Do you have any other worries about you health?

and if necessary,

Anything else?

> ### Key Points
>
> Find out
> - how the patient feels about the problem
> - what aspects of the situation concern the patient
> - how much of a concern they are for the patient

3. Ask patients if they need any more information in addition to that they have already been given.   It remains then to ask if there is any information that the patients want about their condition or treatment, for example:

Is there any part of your illness or treatment that you would like to know about?

Carrying out this simple assessment will help to clearly identify most patient's needs for additional information, clarification or correction of mistaken beliefs.

Assessing children's information needs

Assessing the information needs of children should, under most circumstances, take place with the parent where possible. Assessment of children's needs may also be carried out during an admission or preliminary interview. If the parents express the wish for their child not to be informed, then there needs to be a discussion with the parents about this. Wilkinson (1988) emphasizes the importance of maintaining the child's sense of agency or effectiveness. One way this can be achieved is to give the child choices, where possible. However, this has to be balanced against the needs of the parents to fulfill their parenting roles. Loss of or conflict over these roles can be a major source of stress for as many as one in two parents of hospitalized children (LaMontagne and Pawlak 1990; Carnevale, 1990). How this is achieved is not essentially different than in adults. Consider the following example as part of an admissions interview.

HW: Hello. My name is Susan. What's your name?
Pt: Kevin.
HW: Kevin. Good. What do you think of our ward Kevin?
Pt: (Remains silent.)
HW: If this is your first stay in a hospital, I expect it seems a bit strange and scary.
Pt: (Nods tentatively.)
HW: Would you like me to show you and your mum around, and meet some of the other children here?
Pt: (Nods more vigorously.)
HW: Come on then.

(On return to bedside.)

HW: Now my job here is to help your mum look after you while you're here. I also help to look after other children — Shiela who you just met, and Johnny who isn't here just now. Some children like to help look after themselves. We think that's a good idea. Would you like to help your mum and I look after you?
Pt: Yeah.
HW: One way you can help is to tell us what you want. I could talk to you about how you're doing, tell you the test results? Then we can all decide how we can best get you well again.

Pt: (Nods hesitantly.)

HW: If you'd rather your mum and I decide about those sorts of things, that's fine too. You think about it and tell me what you would like later, OK?

Pt: Uhm, me and my mum?

HW: Yes, of course. When I have something to tell you or to ask you about, I'll talk to both you and your mum together. I think that's a good way of doing it.

Real choice for the child must be based on relevant information. For this reason, it is important that health workers, particularly paediatricians or surgeons, develop a relationship which deserves and retains trust by working directly with the child. The parents are important in facilitating this. Their children trust them, and they know their children best. It may also be beneficial for a key health worker to meet with the whole family including siblings to encourage a sense of involvement for the siblings who can suffer at this time.

It is particularly important to work with an adolescent individually, while retaining contact with the family. Within the context of any family consultation, the adolescent should be given a true choice and decision making role. However, as Wilkinson (1988) points out, the extent to which a young person or child of a given age has the right to refuse parts of a consultation or treatment is a grey area. Despite this, if adolescents are not given the information needed to make choices, they cannot have the semblance of a sense of agency. What shouldn't occur is what happened to a child who needed a hernia repair and awoke from the surgery to find he had also been circumcised. The parents thought it a 'good thing' not to tell him in advance. He was 14 years old.

Techniques for improving recall of information

Can presentation be improved to maximize recall of the most important points? The answer is definitely yes. There are several strategies which substantially improve the recall of information. These strategies are all used at the time of giving verbal information.

Avoidance of jargon

The use of technical terms in communications between practitioners and patients has many problems. Health workers generally need technical precision in communicating with their colleagues, but patients may also use jargon, both medical and otherwise. It is important for practitioners to avoid the use of jargon with patients for the following reasons:

* Patients don't understand.
* Misinterpretation of terms is common.

Health workers spend their working life among colleagues who all use medical, nursing and other health-related terminology. Because everyone else knows what is being talked about in these settings, we may presume a level of knowledge that does not exist in patients. A study investigating patients' understanding of the location of their internal organs (lungs, heart, stomach, liver) found many patients were quite incorrect in their knowledge of the most basic anatomy (Boyle, 1970). If the level of lay knowledge is so low, the level of understanding of technical terms and their nuances is likely to be low also.

Even a minimal use of technical terms can lead to problems. We can illustrate this with the anecdote about a patient told by his surgeon that he needed to have the 'gall-bladder taken out' as it was 'inflamed'. When the patient failed to turn up for admission, he was contacted and asked why he didn't come in to hospital. The patient explained that he didn't want his gall-bladder removed because he didn't want to be incontinent, not realizing the difference between the urinary bladder and gall-bladder. The surgeon had assumed a level of knowledge so basic to a surgeon but not to a lay person, with the result that misunderstanding occurred.

The problem is two-sided. Patients sometimes use medical terms incorrectly, imprecisely or with meanings that are idiosyncratic. A patient may use the term 'depression' for a certain mood, but from a clinical perspective it is unclear whether the patient was feeling low, was severely depressed, or somewhere in between the two. Similarly, patients who use the term 'hypertension' may understand that their blood pressure is 'raised', but whether they understand this to the extent that other health workers do is debatable.

Many biological, medical or nursing terms have very different lay meanings. Take the concept of 'nerves', which for the health worker are anatomical structures. For many working class people, 'nerves' has a different meaning, referring to an anxious emotional state or pattern of behaviour. In other words, nerves can also be a diagnostic label in common use. Similarly, Blumenhagen (1980) reports that the term hypertension was frequently used among the American lay public to denote excessive muscular activity. Whereas many people do not have quite such extreme misinterpretations, the meaning intended by the patient in using a jargon term may not extend to the range of pathology that may both contribute to, or result from, such a diagnosis. Yet when a patient uses a medical term the health worker may be lulled into assuming that the patient and health worker share the same understanding of the term when this will seldom be the case.

Finally, patients may not fully understand the jargon, but feel they should. They thus avoid seeking clarification, fearing ridicule by the health worker or not wishing to appear ignorant.

Thus, use of jargon may lead to both misunderstanding and or assumptions that meaning is shared, when it is not.

Always aim to avoid potential confusion. Where possible use simpler concepts. For example, use high or raised blood pressure instead of hypertension. Alternatively, where no clear common term exists, explain in short, simple terms the nature of the problem. Then give the name. It may also help to write the name on a piece of paper.

Key Points:

Avoid jargon, technical terms, neologisms ('Angio'), initials (D and C, CVA, AMI etc.).

Use instead descriptions in non-technical language. Pitch the level of explanation at the appropriate developmental and educational level.

For children, use very simple terms.

Avoid condescension or implying that the patient should know.

For example:

> Your body can't make enough of a substance called insulin. Because of this, too much sugar stays in your blood. This can make you very sick.
> You need to take insulin to stop you from getting sick.
> We call this diabetes.

This level of explanation avoids technical terms and is very suitable for use with children. Younger children may not fully understand concepts like sugar in blood. An even more basic description may need to be used such as:

Your body uses a food called sugar, and this is what helps you
move and do things.
Sometimes your body can't use the sugar it has.
Then you can get sick.
When this happens, we have to give a very special medicine so
your body can use the sugar again.
We call this medicine insulin.

Order of presentation of material

The second technique to facilitate recall involves how information is presented. This is crucial in understanding and then memorizing information.
If we were discussing a nursing or medical diagnosis, we might talk about
the topic from different perspectives. For example, what the diagnosis is;
what caused it; what can be done about it; what the likely outcome will
be; how it might affect the patient; and what the patient must or must not
do. By the time we have finished talking, we may have ranged across various topics to do with the diagnosis. We have talked about only one
diagnosis, but in a very homogenous fashion. This kind of unstructured
speech has been called amorphous talking. Many points may have been
made but to expect a patient to recall more than a tiny fraction of these is
totally unrealistic as the capacity of working memory is only about 7 ($\pm$2)
units of information. Recall also that memory is creative, often storing what
it is believed to have been the case, rather than what is actually the case.

Research on learning clearly demonstrates that people remember the
beginning and end of a string of presented material far better than they do
the middle section. This primacy and recency effect can be used to advantage in giving information. By placing important information at the
beginning or the end of an information giving session, you can improve
the likelihood of it being recalled.

Key Points

Structure the information you give to patients.

Put important information at the beginning to end of an information-giving session.

Use of emphasis

The third technique uses emphasis to enhance important points. Emphasis identifies information as outstanding, and information that is outstanding is more likely to be recalled than other information. Use statements such as:

> Now, this is very important.
> I want you to pay special attention to . . .

Emphasis makes important information stand out more.

Key Points

Emphasize important points.

Use of repetition

Repetition is a widely used means of trying to improve recall. Parents use it to teach their children, students in studying for exams. All of us use it to retain a telephone number before we write it down. Continuous repetition of information will not make you popular with the patient. Yet, by repeating important information, emphasis can be achieved, thus improving recall.

> Now it's important to take all of the tablets. Remember, take *all* of the tablets.
> I want you to finish the bottle. Don't stop taking them once the symptoms stop.

Key Points

Repeat important information. Remember, repeat important information. Don't forget how important it is to repeat important information.

Explicit categorization

The fifth technique involves organizing information before giving it to the patient. We know that information that is meaningful is more likely to be recalled than information that is not meaningful. Explicit categorization (Ley, 1978) refers to a technique where information for the patient is clearly allocated to meaningfully organized categories. For example, for a patient, these may include 'diagnosis', 'outcome', 'medicine', 'self-treatment', and so on. It is important to clearly outline the categories you intend to use for organizing the material you are going to present *before* you begin to give the information.

> First, I am going to tell you the test results.
> Then I will tell you what is wrong with you.
> Next, I will explain what will happen to you.
> Last, I will tell you what treatment there is.

> First, the test results show that you have an infection deep in your chest, but that is all. That's all I want to say about the tests.
> Second, what is wrong with you. You have a lot of mucous deep in your lungs. This is what makes it difficult for you to breath properly. This is caused by the infection. We call this problem 'pneumonia'. It is a serious condition.
> Now, what will happen to you if we don't treat it is you may get very sick and would eventually be unable to breathe. Fortunately, we can treat the infection very effectively.
> Now, let's talk about the treatment you need. We can soon stop the infection. You will need to take a course of antibiotic medicine. I will also give you some medicine to loosen the mucous in you chest . . . and some more to stop you making much more for a while.

Note that the categories are outlined before they are discussed.

Ley et al (1973) reports an increase of almost 50% in the amount of information recalled when explicit categorization is compared to ordinary presentation.

Key Points

Structure the information you give to patients.

Use explicit categories for presenting information.

Outline the categories before presenting the detailed information in each category at a time.

Specific versus general information

Among the most common types of communication in health care is giving instructions. Instructions may be about medication, or on changing behaviour in some manner. Most of this kind of information is given in very general terms.

> Eat less salt.
> Reduce you intake of fats.
> Try and get more exercise.
> Try and get more rest.
> Don't overdo it.
> Try not to worry so much.

Though indicating *what* should be done, they offer no help in deciding *when* sufficient has been done. They offer no help to the patient in deciding when the *goal* of the instruction has been achieved. The vague nature of the instruction may even generate anxiety in patients over whether or not they are following the instructions correctly. In other patients, the result may be non-adherence.

Many information booklets give data for the patient, but often this is not accompanied by explicit instructions for use. For example, a booklet for post-myocardial infarction patients may usefully contain a list of the cholesterol content of different foods. Yet without specifying the daily ceiling for cholesterol intake, it becomes worse than useless to the patient.

The use of general information is therefore often worse than useless:

> Take plenty of exercise.

How much is plenty? Is this enough? When there is no clear indicator of having achieved the required exercise (in this example), uncertainty makes adherence difficult, even if recall is intact.

By providing specific information, there is both a greater likelihood of recall and more tangible indication of adherence.

Walk for at least 20 minutes every day.

There is a clear 'fact' to be recalled and a clear indication of when the task has been achieved by the patient.

Key Points

Be precise. Don't say to a patient 'Get plenty of exercise'.

Instead say 'Walk at least five miles every day,' or better still, 'Swim at least 30 lengths of the pool three times a week.'

Combining all the above

Combining all the above approaches gives a set of strategies that significantly increase recall of information. Consider the following;

> First, I will tell you how the test will feel. Then I will tell you the purpose of the test. Third I'll tell you what we will be doing to help, and finally, fourth, what you can do to help us and yourself. Then I can answer any questions you might have. How does that sound?
>
> First, what will it feel like? For the test, we need you to swallow a tube into your stomach. The tube is quite thin. It will go down easily. It may make you gag a bit. You will be awake because you need to swallow when we ask you to. It might feel a bit strange, but will not be painful.
>
> Now I want to talk about why we're doing this test. We want to have a look at the inside of your stomach to see if there is any obvious cause for your stomach pains. The tube you will swallow lets us look into your stomach. That way we don't need to do an operation. The test itself lasts for about 20 minutes.
>
> Now, third, let's talk about what you can do to help, and what we will do. Now it is important you remember this, OK? Remember, we will give you some medicine to help you swallow

the tube. Remember I said you need to help? When you are told to do so, you must swallow hard to help get the tube into your stomach. Remember to keep swallowing hard until I tell you to stop. That's it.

So, to summarize, first you will be swallowing a tube through which we can look into your stomach. Second, it will make you gag a bit, but when that happens, you should swallow hard and that will help the tube go down, and third, we will give you a sedative to minimise any gagging.

Do you have any questions?

This example serves to illustrate how material can be organized to make use of order of presentation, emphasis, repetition, and explicit categorization. Material presented in this way will be easier for the patient to recall than if the same material were presented without formal structure.

Key Points

To maximize patient recall of information combine the following techniques:
- avoidance of jargon
- presenting important material at the beginning and end
- use of emphasis for important points
- use of repetition
- use of explicit categorization
- use of specific rather than general instructions

Use of written and other types of information

Sometimes, complex information has to be given to patients, or patients need to carry out careful preparation for certain tests, such as colonoscopy. In this case, providing written information can greatly assist recall of detail. Many organizations, self-help groups and special interest groups now produce detailed information booklets for patients. These can be obtained from organizations such as the British Heart Foundation for cardiac diseases, The Imperial Cancer Research Fund, for leaflets on different types of cancer, the American Diabetic Association, and so forth.

It is important where such information sheets are produced locally, that they should be understandable by 80% or more of the population. This has not always been the case. Ley et al found in the early 1970s that most X-ray information leaflets issued by a hospital serving a lower working class area were too difficult for the intended patients to understand. Other studies have reported similar findings (Evans, 1968; Ley, 1978).

More recently, audio tapes have been used to record disclosure of information during consultations with patients having cancer for the patient's later use. The patient can play the information back later to clarify points of misunderstanding. This can also help the patient having to explain many times to relatives; the tape can be given to the relative instead. This was rated as helpful by 100% of 39 patients who listened to tapes as part of an evaluative study of taped disclosure. A further 15/39 patients said the tape contained information which they had forgotten following the consultation. Only 21% (8/39) of patients found the tapes upsetting despite the frankness of discussion they contained (Hogbin and Fallowfield, 1989).

Other means of information giving have been explored, including using computer data points for access to medical information contained on intelligent health records (Jones et al, 1990). These will not be discussed further here. Clearly, however, there is much innovation in attempts to improve patient access to information. However, the first line of information giving remains first and foremost the responsibility of the health worker.

Summary

- Most patients don't get as much information as they want.
- Even when efforts are made to give information, much is not recalled and satisfaction remains low.
- Much non-adherence of instructions is either due to patients not understanding or not remembering information.
- Jargon on both sides leads to misunderstandings.
- Disorganized presentation (amorphous talking) is largely wasted breath.
- Vague and general instructions are not easy to remember and difficult to follow.
- Take the patient's health beliefs into account.
- Effective technique includes:
  - avoidance of jargon

- presenting important material at the beginning and end
- use of emphasis for important points
- use of repetition
- use of explicit categorization
- use of specific rather than general instructions.

Exercises

1. *You are the health worker.*   Your (adult) patient is soon to be discharged from hospital following an acute respiratory infection. The patient has chronic obstructive airways disease, and a history of asthma compounded by smoking. Your task is to explain to the patient the diagnosis and the etiology of the condition (why the patient was admitted to hospital). If is also important that the patient stop smoking and take regular daily gentle exercise; swimming would be particularly beneficial, and uses medication and an inhaler appropriately. Medication side-effects are occasional but can include sleep disturbance. The patient is to come for an outpatient visit in two weeks time.

    You are the patient.   (Be your own age and sex.) You have been in hospital with a chest infection. The staff have told you to give up smoking. You have tried before but didn't succeed. You have asthma, and are afraid to take exercise in case it causes an asthma attack. You are eager to get home once again.

    Five minutes after the role-play ends, the 'patient' should be asked to write down all the information that can be recalled from the role play.

    How much information was recalled?

2. *You are the health worker.*   You are involved in the discharge of a patient from hospital. The patient has been diagnosed and treated for insulin-dependent diabetes mellitus. (There is a problem with the production of insulin, without which the cells of the body cannot use glucose. Excesses of glucose can accumulate causing the patient to lose consciousness. Insulin has to be replaced in correct amount to meet the needs of glucose level in blood so that the cells of the body can use glucose.) The patient is stable and has been told of the diagnosis. Your task is to instruct the patient in self-care. This involves the following:

Inject insulin daily, to be altered to accommodate exercise and stress (increase amount injected by 10–20 units/day). Maintain steady fluid intake. Avoid concentrated carbohydrates, such as sugar, chocolates, etc., eating an equivalent amount per day in terms of energy content, and eventually, regulating insulin use to match dietary changes. Check glucose level daily using of urinary glucose/ blood glucose measurement (choose one). Visit out-patient clinic once every three months.

You are also to give any other information you feel the patient needs at the time of interview. Use the recommended strategy for giving information.

You are the patient. (Be yourself as much as possible.) You have been in hospital for eight days following a blackout. You were found to have diabetes. You are not sure what this is, though you have heard of the condition. You are to be discharged from hospital later today. When you have your interview, ask for an explanation of the condition, what you need to do, and what treatment you will be given.

Five minutes after the role-play ends, the 'patient' should be asked to write down all the information that can be recalled from the role play.

How much information was recalled?

Discussion

1. What are the advantages of using the recommended strategy for information giving?

2. Even with the recommended strategy for information giving, much information will be forgotten. What else can be done to increase patient recall of information?

3. What preliminary enquiries should be made before giving information to the patient, and why?

4. You are responsible for developing written material introducing a common procedure undertaken in your unit, which will be given to patients to help prepare them for the procedure. Discuss what needs to be considered in producing this material.

5. Consider the advantages and disadvantages of introducing a programme for tape-recording information-giving sessions for patients, in order that the patients have a better record of what was said to them.

10

Handling Difficult Questions

Educational Objectives

By the end of this chapter , you should be able to

- give three or more reasons to explain why health workers avoid handling difficult questions
- recognize and avoid appropriate and inappropriate use of re-assurance
- recognize common avoidance tactics to questions
- recognize the value of assessing patients' information requirements and basing information giving on that assessment
- demonstrate at least one approach to assessing information needs
- recognize the value of a clearly understood unit policy for handling difficult questions
- describe strategies for dealing with uncertainty
- describe the role of reflective questions in the assessment of patients' information needs
- recognize the place of timely and appropriate reassurance
- recognize that when patients ask for information they almost always expect to be told the truth

Introduction

Most of us know what it is like to be asked a difficult question. For children and adults, difficult questions are a source of discomfort and even anxiety. The fact that some difficult questions are innocent, as when children ask about their origins, or why their pet died, seldom make them easier to answer than questions such as 'Have I got cancer?'. Difficult questions are difficult because they may seem to pose a threat to either the questioner or the questioned, or both. For example, being asked if you were responsible for a treatment omission implies the threat of discipline for negligence or breach of tort. Another example is when we know our answer will cause pain to another. In this case, and others, there seems to be a tendency to avoid honest answers, preferring instead to comfort, reassure or avoid answering at all.

Common reasons for avoidance

For a health worker who may be asked some very difficult questions by patients, a common response is to avoid the issue. This has been shown to occur extensively in health care (Maguire, 1985). At least three sets of reasons can be identified for avoiding difficult questions in health care settings.

Role boundaries

The first reason arises from perceptions of professional role responsibilities. To many health workers, traditional role boundaries are not to be crossed. Thus, doctors diagnose and plan treatment, nurses provide physical care, physiotherapists maintain mobility, pharmacists provide medication, and occupational therapists contribute to rehabilitation. When it comes to answering difficult questions, most other health workers perceive it to be the doctor's job. This may be seen as a blessing in disguise for the non-medical health worker who thereby avoids a difficult situation.

Acknowledging the professional role of nurses and other practitioner groups as providers of information in response to patient questions removes some of the responsibility (and some of the control) from the medical profession. Nonetheless, there are still certain types of information that patients prefer to receive from their doctors. Specifically, information on diagnosis and prognosis and on treatment was reportedly *preferred* from doctors rather than from others, whereas supportive and emotional care was seen as more *likely* from nursing sources (French, 1979). However, with the increases in nursing specialization, more nurses are becoming knowledgeable in treatment areas in their own right and this preference for sources of information may be changing. Many experienced nurses are in a better position than a newly qualified house officer to answer patients' questions on diagnosis.

Though patients seem to prefer certain types of information from certain health workers (French, 1979), not all patients respect these professional roles to the same extent. Moreover, if the preferred information source is unavailable an alternative source will be asked. Patients may ask the occupational therapist about their medical treatment, a nurse about their future mobility, or the pharmacist about return to work. In contrast, while the health worker may like to give a straight answer to the patient, many believe it is 'not their job' to be the one to give the particular information requested. Hence, nurses (and most other professional groups) traditionally respond to difficult questions from a patient by saying something like:

> You'll have to ask Doctor about that.

or,

> Would you like to talk to Doctor Man?

or,

> I'm not sure, I'll ask someone to come and have a word.

Junior nurses and junior medical staff may in turn be inhibited from acting independently in response to the demands of the situation in case they 'let the cat out of the bag' and get into trouble. The senior medical staff and experienced ward nurse may have acquired a range of skilled avoidance responses for dealing with particularly awkward questions.

Not upsetting the patient

A second reason why difficult questions by patients may not get answered has to do with a general unwillingness by health workers to say things which may 'upset' patients. Causing upset to patients seems to be considered almost criminal by some health workers. This concern for the patients' feelings is commendable. However, given that the emotional dimension of ill-health is otherwise rarely considered one might be forgiven for the slightly cynical view that this sudden concern is more for staff than patient benefit. A more basic reason seems to involve anxiety on the part of the health workers about causing upset. Many health workers worry that if they answer a patient honestly, and the news is bad, then some unforeseen collapse of the patient will occur and the health workers cannot cope. This catastrophic thinking is enough to discourage direct responses to difficult questions. (See also Chapter 11 for a fuller discussion of this point.)

Lack of skill in disclosure

The third and perhaps most fundamental reason is that most health workers don't know how to handle the difficult questions asked by patients. This is not surprising. Telling people they have AIDS, or that their child, spouse or parent is seriously ill is difficult. For that reason alone, it is important that such questions be handled with care and sensitivity.

The result of these strategies for patients is that their questions are often left unanswered or are given only partial or vague replies. As in other situations, the uncertainty caused by this often generates more problems than it solves.

This chapter explores ways to handle difficult questions effectively.

Whose illness is it anyway? Openness versus secrecy

Difficult questions in health care come in many different forms. When answers are given, the questioners (patients or relatives) can better appraise their situation. Avoiding difficult questions has the opposite effect. It reduces the questioners' resources for accurate appraisal, thereby increasing uncertainty.

Children's rights to answers

There may be even greater unwillingness on the part of staff to answer difficult questions from children. Children are ascribed fewer rights than adults to information and involvement in their care. They also tend to be less skilled at asking questions and more discouraged by non-verbal and contextual factors. Though now somewhat archaic, the phrase 'Children should speak when they're spoken to' exemplifies their (continued) low status in society. Thus, children may be even further removed from access to the information they want than adults.

Parents and medical staff are generally unwilling to abrogate their parental or professional control by allowing children a voice in what is done to them in the name of health care (Lewis and Lewis, 1990). However, allowing the child this participation can prove beneficial to the child (Hart-Zeldin, Kalnins, Pollack and Love, 1990; Lewis and Lewis, 1990).

Adolescence

Young adolescents of 12 or 13 years old are different to those of 15 years old, who are different again to those of 17 or 18 years old. Nonetheless, health workers may answer the questions of adolescents the same way as for young children. Yet adolescents are not young children. Older adolescents may be more forceful in their requests, while younger ones may demonstrate sullenness or uncooperativeness, perhaps in the form of non-adherence to treatment or diet as a means of protesting their powerlessness. Having just graduated from childhood, it is likely many are unwilling to return to their former dependency. Common complaints of adolescents about adult health workers are that they are not listened to by the health worker; that health workers always side with the parent; that the adolescent is patronized by health workers; that there is misunderstanding (probably on both sides) about the questions being asked; that adults are nosy; and that adults lack a sense of humour (Wrate, 1989).

Common responses for avoiding difficult questions

Below are some responses for avoiding difficult questions likely to be seen in clinical practice. How often have you used these or similar strategies?

Reassurance

A question may generate immediate reassurance from the health worker, enabling the health worker to avoid dealing with the issues raised by the question. This may happen when the question indicates patient anxiety, awareness of a problem, or when health workers want to avoid discussing a subject they are unsure about. Reassurance is probably the most common response to expressions of emotion.

Pt: Am I going to be in hospital long?
HW: Now don't you worry. We'll have you out as soon as possible.
Pt: I don't think I'll be able to manage this colostomy.
HW: Most people manage fine after they get used to it.
Pt: I don't think I can get used to this.
HW: Oh yes you will, it just takes time . . .

This kind of response may be especially common when the patient is a child or adolescent. (See Chapter 8 for further discussion of this problem.)

Changing the subject or pretending not to hear

Another way of avoiding difficult issues raised by patients' questions is by failing to acknowledge the question. As two people are needed for a conversation to succeed, when one party refuses to pick up the conversation, it cannot take place. A common form of this occurs when one person hides behind a stream of words.

Pt: Will it be painful?
HW: We do hundreds of these operations every year and all the patients I've nursed have no problems. Is anyone coming to visit you today?
Pt: What I don't understand is why I have to have these tests done?
HW: Have you ever been in hospital before?
Pt: Is everything all right?
HW: When did you last have a checkup?

It can be difficult to respond this way as to do so requires more social distance. One has to be particularly immune to social pressure to use this approach. Most staff try to be warm and supportive to patients where possible, making reassurance or avoidance a more likely response.

Straightforward avoidance

Avoidance comes in many forms. These range from apparently simple oversights or failure to pick up cues given by the patient through to 'urgent' telephone calls that have to be made immediately. More direct avoidance includes getting 'someone else to tell you about that', and so forth.

Pt: Is it something serious?
HW: (to another) Can you see that these tests get done before the weekend — Don't worry we'll soon have you right.

Pt: Is my father going to be all right?
HW: Excuse me, I have to answer my pager. I'll be back in a moment.

Pt: I'm glad to be going home. What were the results?
HW: I'll be writing to your GP and he'll fill you in on the details.

The desire for information

There are many variants on strategies for avoiding difficult questions. People can be very creative. One important question that remains unanswered, however, is *should* patients be given answers to their questions. It bears repetition that studies examining patients' desire for information, almost without exception, show 80% to 90% of patients want as much information as possible about their illness, even if the news is bad (Blanchard et al, 1988). This is a consistent finding. This point is raised several times throughout this book because it is important and yet so often overlooked. Try this simple exercise. Ask the class or group to which you belong the following questions.

How many of you would tell your patients if they had cancer? About 30% to 50% might raise their hands. Now ask: 'If you had a serious illness, such as cancer, raise your hand if you would want to be told about it.' More than 80% of the group asked are likely to raise their hands.

In order to improve the provision of information to patients in response to 'difficult' questions, we need to acknowledge several important points.

The desire for ignorance

It would be wrong to suggest that all patients want to know everything about all aspects of their illness. Some patients do not want to know the details. Some want the health workers to make the decisions about their care. Some, a few, do not want to know their diagnosis, preferring instead to deny their condition. It must be emphasized that though such patients are in the minority, this is no reason to treat their wishes differently from those of the majority. If they ask questions, they deserve the respect of a considered answer.

On first sight, this poses a problem. How does the health worker decide what kind of answer the patient wants? Of course, we might assume that all patients want good news — for their fears to be refuted by the health worker. Yet, in principle, there should only be one answer to questions — the truth. Most patients want honest and realistic answers to their questions in order that they might make informed decisions. Some, however, might not be ready for the enormity of the answer they will receive. It is important, therefore, for health workers to be sensitive to these needs and to develop a policy of handling difficult questions appropriately and effectively. In this way they are prepared to give appropriate details to meet the patient's current needs.

Key Points

Patients *want* information on their condition, even if that information might be upsetting.

The majority of patients who are given upsetting information can 'take it', even though they may be appropriately upset as a result.

Some patients do react badly, but with time and support, they can and do cope.

Patients have a right to information about their condition.

Patients should be allowed and encouraged to participate in decision making about their own illness.

Patients need accurate information if they are to make informed decisions regarding their health and treatment.

Questions tend to be asked because answers are wanted. Deciding for the patient removes power and responsibility from them, and as such is a political act.

The problem of not getting answers to questions

A major difficulty for patients is getting information upon which to make informed decisions. For example, it is not uncommon for patients and their relatives to be shunted between different practitioners, specialists, wards and units (Thorne, 1993). There may be many different professionals involved in the patient's care during the course of an illness. Under such circumstances, responsibility for overall care of the patient and family can become diffuse. No one may take responsibility for the whole patient, though each may take responsibility for a different part or aspect of treatment. When this happens, who does the patient ask? When specialists are asked about an area other than their own, they may be unable or unwilling to comment on what is seen as someone else's specialty. Nursing staff and junior medical staff may not answer questions for fear of ignorance. At visiting time, patients' relatives may be unable to find a health worker to ask questions, either for themselves or on behalf of the patients. Family physicians seldom visit their patients during their stay in hospital, and if they hear the hospitalization details, it is after discharge. So the GP can rarely help.

Where loose multidisciplinary team care exists, there is a greater tendency to assume that someone else will tell or has told the patient all the required information. This, sadly, all too often does not happen. For multidisciplinary care to be effective it needs to rely on a high level of communications between different team members that is usually lacking.

Similar problems can occur in out-patient settings. Patients may feel unwilling to press their practitioners for information for fear of being perceived as 'difficult' or 'neurotic'. Many patients collude with the traditional power hierarchy of practitioner-patient, feeling they will be told what they need to know (Wilkinson, 1988). Nurses may feel unwilling to give additional information to a patient without first consulting a doctor. There is seldom a unit policy for clarifying who is responsible for answering patients' questions.

There is one other reason why patients' questions may not be answered. It is common for health workers to be asked questions that they cannot answer. But rather than admit that they don't know, some health workers will unconsciously continue to maintain the illusion of professional omnipotence, that they know all aspects of the patient's treatment and prognosis, when in fact they do not. Others just don't like to say 'I don't know', feeling they somehow fail the patient. However, most patients would appreciate this admission. It reveals the health worker to be more human and accessible.

Consequently, special attention needs to be given to providing appropriate answers to patients' questions.

It would be unduly pessimistic to argue that no information is given to patients about their illness and treatment. Many health workers try hard to give effective information to patients. The focus of this chapter is that patients find it hard to obtain information on difficult subjects.

So far, questions are considered difficult if the answer would be hard for the patient/relative to cope with. But there are other types of difficult questions, for example why certain things were or were not done during a course of treatment. There are questions or accusations of substandard care which are, unfortunately, becoming increasingly common. People expect better standards of service, and many are not satisfied with bland reassurances that flow too easily off the tongue.

Recently, a woman was awarded damages of over £400 000 by the UK courts for incompetent emergency care received by her husband following a riding accident. This case illustrates how difficult it can be for a lay person to obtain accurate information on cases of suspected negligence or less-than-adequate care. Health workers confronted with a question about an aspect of care may feel that their professional competence is being challenged. When gross negligence or malpractice is apparent, or a sudden unexpected bad outcome arises, patients or relatives may not realize how threatening repeated questions about treatment or care may appear to the health worker. When unexplained problems in patient care do arise, staff may become very defensive in response to questions. Most health workers are aware that mistakes do occur in hospital care.

Problems faced by children and adolescents

Children and adolescents have less status and therefore less power within our societies. Their rights to be treated as individuals and to expect honest replies to their questions are compromised by paternalistic tendencies as adults to 'protect' them from harm. In many countries, the law requires that children and young people under the age of 17 or 18 be considered minors, and consequently that health care staff act *in loco parentis* to see that they come to no harm.

This legal responsibility can be an additional barrier to children having difficult questions answered. Discussion with parents on how to respond to difficult questions may not fully prepare the health worker for the often penetrating innocent questions a child can ask.

Health workers are often unwilling to give information considered 'difficult' to adults. Health workers, especially physicians (Lewis and Lewis, 1990) are even more unwilling to give such information to children. This remains the case despite the fact that evidence suggests children are at least as capable as adults in adapting to the implications of ill health (Lewis and Lewis, 1990).

For children then, the parent may be kept informed. But even this can be problematic if the child's condition is serious, or the prognosis poor and protective parental responses predominate. It may be virtually impossible for a child to get information from staff unwilling to bypass the parent, or from parents concerned to protect their child from the upsetting truth.

All of the strategies used to avoid dealing with difficult questions, whether from children or adults, result in the need to further withhold information or avoid dealing with issues.

▰ Reflecting questions back to clients

Minimizing the risk of patients not receiving appropriate answers to difficult questions involves reflection. Reflection has already been mentioned in previous chapters and will only be briefly reiterated here with examples.

The aim of the technique is to re-present, or reflect the question back to the patient before answering in full. The following excerpt from a discussion between a health worker and the parents of a young girl comatose following a closed head injury serves as an example:

Rel: Will our daughter be all right when she regains consciousness?

HW: Yes, well I'll answer your question. Could you tell me why you ask? It would help me to answer you more fully.

Rel: I've heard of people being really badly affected after head injuries, you know. We're frightened that she won't be able to look after herself when she's recovered.

HW: You think that will happen with your daughter?

Rel: Well, yes, we're frightened that she will need a lot of looking after, be, er, . . . handicapped, and we . . . , we both work you see.

HW: I can see it must be a big worry for you. Well, I'm afraid we won't know until she comes around how much she has been affected. Though she may recover very quickly, I must warn you I'm afraid most people with similar injuries take many months before they are recovered. What we do know is the sooner she regains conscious, the less extensive any brain damage might be.

Rel: What will she . . . ? How will it affect her?

HW: That's difficult to say. She may have difficulty with her memory, not be able to concentrate, but we won't really know until she wakes up. Until then I wouldn't like to say really.

In the above example, the first reflection unearths information about why the parent is concerned. In some cases, concern for the well being of the patient may seem obvious. But there may be other reasons for the question that the reflective response can identify. By asking 'Do you think that will happen to your daughter?' the health worker identifies the parental anxiety regarding caring for a head injured daughter. This is also useful for the information it gives about the parents' acceptance that head injuries do often have lasting consequences. Such information may be of use later when discussing any residual impairment. The issue of impairment might then be dealt with more easily when the time comes. This helps prepare the parents for what could be otherwise devastating bad news later on.

The health worker could have offered reassurance, which would have been unrealistic given the possible extent of the injury, and would likely have made coping with the reality of the situation more difficult later if the patient did have severe residual impairment.

The health worker could say, 'We won't know until she regains consciousness'. But this would not have identified the concerns of the questioner. These concerns may indicate both how the parents are coping, and also unanticipated problems associated with care of the patient. Thus, in using reflection, the health worker was able to first gather information on the motivation for the question, and from there make an appropriate yet honest answer. Using this approach can increase the health worker's sense of control over the situation while meeting the parents' needs.

In the same way that information increases the ability of the staff to cope with the patient, it also increases the ability of patients and relatives to cope.

▦ Responding to the question

Younger children

It is important to reiterate that in answering difficult questions, responses should always be as non-technical as possible. In the case of children, responses should be at a language level appropriate to their intellectual development.

In addition to the problems adults have of getting straight answers to their questions, children may not understand they have the right to ask questions. It is important then that they be 'given permission' to ask questions in a way they can understand. By letting them know they can, you give them permission. This removes one moral prohibition that may hinder their asking questions.

Make a clear and unambiguous statement that you are willing to answer any questions they may have.

> I expect it's a bit scary not knowing what's going on. If you like we can talk about it.
> Shall I tell you what we want to do to make you better?

It is important to demonstrate a sincerely empathic attitude to the child. Younger children usually benefit from having the main caretaker or both parents present at the time. Even uniformed health workers can be frightening to a four-year-old. Of course, children younger than four should have a caretaker with them throughout their period of hospitalization. For older children, a talk with the parents first will probably take place. However, it is important that the health worker explain the importance of honesty to the child and encourages the parents to be open.

An empathic approach may help the child to formulate the question they cannot put into words.

> I expect you want to know what's wrong, do you?

Avoid complex terms or sentence structures (e.g. double negatives).

Pause frequently to give time for the child to digest what is being said. Children may take a long time to think about what is being said to them.

Key Points

Use short and simple sentences.

Pause frequently.

Avoid complex or technical terms.

Pt: Am I going to die?

HW: That's a very big question. It's very difficult to answer. I'll try to explain, so stop me if you don't understand, OK?

(Pause.)

Pt: OK.

HW: You have two kidneys. One here and one here (points). Their job is to clean the blood. When they don't work, it causes all sorts of problems.

(Pause.)

Pt: What kind of problems?

HW: Well, the most important problem is they don't clean your blood anymore. So you become sick from all the waste that builds up in your blood. This would normally be removed in your urine.

(Pause.)

Also, your kidneys remove any water your body doesn't need. When they don't work, your body keeps too much water, so you get all puffy. Then you have to be careful about how much you drink.

Pt: Can't I drink when I get thirsty?

HW: Yes, but maybe not as much as you could before.

(Long pause.)

HW: Would you like me to tell you about what we do to help these problems go away?. . .

Adolescents and older children

Reflective questions are one way of handling questions from adolescents and children over ten years of age. It is important to bear in mind that most young people appear to have the intellectual ability to deal with such questions. Emotionally, however, they often lack the experience to cope in an adult way and may need greater support while feeling unwilling to allow themselves to become dependent (Wrate, 1988). There are differences between children and adults: it may be more difficult for some young people to identify or admit their feelings and motivations in an open way. Many adults can have this difficulty too, so it is hardly surprising that young people do.

Adolescents may also have more difficulty relating in a comfortable way with health workers. The establishment of a good relationship with the patient is therefore a priority.

Treating adolescents in a sincere way as people with their own choices is important here. Being prepared to admit mistakes also makes the health worker human and more trustworthy (Wrate, 1988).

For other children, there may be a greater straightforwardness both in their questions and their expectation of answers. A second point is that people, children included, can and do vary tremendously in their emotional maturity for any given age. One 12-year-old girl might be more emotionally mature in terms of self-confidence and in relationships with adults than, say, a boy of 16. Chronological age is no guarantee of maturity, but neither should it be an excuse to avoid difficult questions.

Key Points

For adolescents,
- establish a relationship
- let them know you are willing to discuss any questions they might have
- be prepared to spend the time doing this
- treat the adolescent as a person, not a child
- be sincere and honest
- use simple sentences, avoiding complex sentences and technical terms
- have an (appropriate) sense of humour

Handling adults' questions

There is a range of difficult questions that adults will ask. Questions about diagnosis, and the nature of treatment can usually be answered by health workers. Questions about treatment outcome, prognoses and causes are more difficult to answer, and may be unknown. Finally, questions about patient or staff behaviour, policy or practice may challenge skills or treatment approaches. These may be more personal and threatening to health workers.

Diagnosis and treatment

Difficult questions about diagnosis and treatment seldom arise if a policy of involving the patient in decision making and open information is used. However, there will be situations where difficult questions arise. These almost always involve disclosing bad news. For example, to the mother of a stillborn child; to the parents or the child with cancer; to the patient with incurable illness. As such, these issues will be dealt with in the next chapter: Breaking Bad News.

Treatment outcome, prognoses and causes

Difficult questions are often difficult because of the uncertainty they embody which the health worker cannot control. These situations often involve the efficacy of treatment, the prognosis (outcome) of a disease, and the cause of a problem or illness. A moment's thought reveals the uncertain nature of these issues. When asked to answer such questions, the health worker is, in effect, being asked to predict the future or speculate about imponderables, something few can do with certainty.

Pt: If I have the operation, will I be cured?

HW: Er . . . ., well, that's a very difficult question to answer. If by cure you mean being free from the disease forever, then no one can guarantee that.

Pt: But you're asking me to agree to have my leg cut off, . . . and you're saying it's not going to cure me?

HW: No. What I said was there's no guarantee. What I can say is that of 100 people with this disease who have this operation, 65 of them will still be free from the disease in five years' time.

Pt: So you're saying that I have a 65% chance of being OK for only five years? That doesn't sound like very good odds to me. That means there's a 35% chance that the disease will come back. And within five years, even if I have my leg cut off!

HW: If you have the operation there is one chance in three of recurrence. If you don't have the operation the, er . . . , treatment alternatives are very few, and you will almost certainly not survive five years.

Pt: Some choice.

HW: It's a very difficult decision we have to make. I'm sorry I can't be more positive. It would be wrong of me to mislead you. The one thing I can say is the one-in-three figure is for treatments done five or six years ago. We think we're doing better now, so those odds may be better too. I wish I could offer you something more certain.

Pt: Yeah, well . . . I, I need to think it over.

This kind of situation is one of the most difficult to deal with. A young adult with a life threatening disease, requiring aggressive mutilative surgery, with an uncertain prognosis asks the question 'If I agree to this, will I be cured?' There might be a tendency to say yes. (Many medical opinions consider being disease free for five years equivalent to a cure; most patients consider cure to be lifelong freedom from recurrence, which for a young adult may be 30 to 50 years.) In this example, the health worker correctly clarifies any misunderstanding about what can be expected from the treatment in an honest and sensitive manner.

Questions about causality can also be difficult to handle. For example the parent of a comatose adolescent admitted following an heroin overdose presents a double shock to the parents who were unaware of their child's drug habit.

Parent: How long will he be like this?

HW: Well, we've given him an antidote, to counter the heroin. For the time being he's stable. He's now breathing on his own; that's a good sign. We should know in a couple of hours if he's going to come around.

Parent: Why would he do this? This isn't John!

HW: You didn't know he used drugs?

Parent: No, he would never . . . He was cheerful. His school work was good; he'd decided to go to university . . .

HW: Sometimes young people don't know what they're injecting. It's quite a common problem in this town.

Parent: But why would he do something . . . , use that stuff?

HW: I can't tell you why. I don't know. Let's wait and see how he recovers.

The parents were having difficulties accepting not just the patient's coma, but additionally the shock of realizing he had a heroin habit. Note how the health worker drops a clear verbal cue about the uncertainty of the patient's recovery: . . . *'if he's going to come around.'* The parent does not pick this up, suggesting that they might not be ready to deal with this at present. The health worker ends by saying 'Let's wait and see', recognizing the parent may be at their coping limit, temporarily withholding discussion of the patient's uncertain prognosis. The health worker is also not afraid to admit ignorance of why the overdose was taken, thereby avoiding further pressure to provide answers the health worker does not have.

A final example of handling a difficult question involves a discussion with the wife of a middle-aged father of ten-year-old twin boys. The woman's husband was diagnosed with pneumonia, and investigations indicated that he was HIV positive. The wife talks with a health visitor.

Pt: I suppose I'm having trouble coming to terms with . . . um . . . what he must have done, been doing. I used to think he wasn't like other husbands, you know, going with other women. I never thought of anything else . . . .

HW: It's a shock.

Pt: I mean, how's it gonna affect us, the boys? What do I tell people when they ask what wrong with him? I can't . . . tell them.

HW: Well, he has pneumonia. That's all you need to say.

Pt: I could kill him! It's not fair on us. What about the boys? I've got to think about them. I don't want him giving it to them. How . . . ? What can I do?

HW: There isn't much risk to you or your boys if you take a few simple hygiene precautions. I can tell you about that. It's not very easy to give HIV to anther person casually. I can see you're very angry with him, and perhaps a bit scared too. Do you want to talk about that?

This example has no single question to handle, but rather a multitude of them. The wife is angry at her husband's assumed infidelity, at the risk posed to her and her children by her husband's behaviour. Many of these difficult questions are rhetorical, not requiring an answer. But some are in need of answering and the health visitor is trying to pick out the issues that seem most urgent. While the husband remains in hospital, risk of transmission is not important, but keeping the family together is. More practical questions like what to tell inquisitive neigbours, and motives for her husband's behaviour are most pressing to this woman at this stage.

A final example illustrates a difficult question directed at the management of an elderly patient by a relative. This kind of situation can generate defensive responses in the staff member if there is some accusation needing to be dealt with.

Rel: Are you in charge?

HW: At the moment, yes. Can I help?

Rel: It's about my mother, Mrs Smith. She said she was, . . . she's quite upset. She told me that she was left naked and in full view of the ward this morning while her bed was being made. Do you know anything about this?

HW: No I didn't, but it certainly is unacceptable if it did happen.

Rel: Well I think it's terrible that this happens. What are there curtains for?

HW: I will talk to the staff who were on duty this morning and the nurse who changed your mother's bed. I'm on duty tomorrow morning. Will you be visiting then?

Rel: I'll be here.

HW: I should be able to explain what happened then. Would that be all right? Meanwhile, I'll remind all the nurses, though I'm sure they have been careful about privacy, they usually are.

Rel: Not according to my mother.

HW: I'll also talk with your mother to find out exactly what happened.

Rel: Thank you.

The unit manager could have responded in a defensive fashion here which may have made future dealings between staff, patient and relative fractious and strained. Accepting the relative's grounds for complaint as potentially legitimate and being prepared to look into the incident disarms any potential aggressiveness. However, in so doing, the unit manager is careful not to accept at face value that the incident occurred as presented. The three examples above are illustrative only. They show a range of clinical situations that can arise in which difficult questions may be presented to the staff.

Giving reassurance

If there is one thing given more than medication in the presence of the sick, it must be reassurance. The one thing given more than anything else in response to difficult questions must be reassurance. Reassurance has been reputed to cure the most intractable conditions, though has seldom been reliably documented as so doing. Like a smile, reassurance apparently costs nothing to administer. When all else fails, reassurance remains available.

And of course, there are those who want to be reassured, and for such, it meets their needs. Perhaps for these reasons, it is so widespread.

Reassurance does have a place, when appropriate, usually after the main issues have been dealt with. For example, patients who have asked why they gain weight and been told that they have a renal problem are likely to have many further questions. Reassuring them that 'everything will be all right' is not going to help if everything is not all right. The range of meanings that even a minor illness may have for a patient is seldom considered by health workers. So it is important that reassurance, when it is given, is both *timely* and *appropriate*.

Reassurance must be timely in that it should be given at the appropriate point in the discussion. There is no rule that can be used to work out when this will be, other than being sensitive to cues the patient is communicating to you and those you are communicating to the patient.

For example, a health worker says:

> The bad news is you have diabetes. The good news is, with your cooperation, we can keep you well for decades.

Even though this may be the truth, the health worker is showing personal insecurity or professional pride rather than offering support to the patient.

Look at another example:

> You have diabetes. It's quite a serious condition. That's the bad news. The good news is that we understand the condition very well, and so many people keep it under control successfully. You will probably need to make some changes in the way you lead you life in order to do so.

This is more realistic. Reassurance is tempered with honest but balanced evaluation of what is required.

Key Points

Consider the meaning of the information to the patient. Discuss this wherever possible.

Give appropriate reassurance at the **time** when it will be effective. Assess this by careful attention to patient cues.

Be honest and realistic in the reassurance you offer.

Remember that it is important for the health worker to understand the meaning that is heard by the patient. This helps to achieve empathy with the patient. Then, understanding when reassurance is appropriate may be more likely to occur much more spontaneously. Listen to what the patient is saying.

When reassurance is given, it should be appropriate in what it is offering. In other words, be realistic. Patients who have just learned they have a chronic degenerative condition like diabetes, or renal disease will not be reassured that 'it's all right'. For them, perhaps, they will never be *all right* again. This is where sensitivity to understanding of the meaning the answer has for the patient comes in. However, the health worker who offers continued care and support for as long as the patient needs it will be providing a more appropriate and effective reassurance.

Summary

When patients ask for information, they expect to be told the truth.

Avoidance of difficult questions is commonly achieved by:
- providing reassurance
- changing the subject
- pretending not to hear the question
- ignoring the question
- avoiding/escaping from the situation

The majority of patients want to know as much as possible about their condition, even if the news is bad:
- Patients want information on their condition, even if that information might be upsetting.
- The majority of patients who are given information can 'take it', even though they may be appropriately upset.
- A minority of patients do react badly, but with time and support, they can and do cope.
- Patients have a right to information about their condition.
- Children and adolescents also have such a right.
- Patients should be allowed and encouraged to participate in decision making about their own illness.
- Patients need accurate information if they are to make informed decisions regarding their health and treatment.

Use reflective questions to decide how much patients want to know.

Use reassurance, but circumspectly.

Exercises

Again, these exercises take the form of role-play dyadic experiences which aim to give provisional experience in alternative ways of handling difficult questions.

1. *Situation:* An middle-aged male has just been admitted following unexpected and sudden loss of consciousness. The patient has no significant medical history. He is accompanied to the hospital by his daughter/son (the relative).
   Task: To discuss the possible implications of the problem in response to questions from the accompanying relative.
   Time available: 5–10 minutes.

   You are the relative.   (Be yourself as much as possible.) Imagine your father has been admitted to hospital following unexpected loss of consciousness. He has no previous history of any serious illness. You are worried that he may have had a stroke and will be handicapped as a result. Put questions voicing your anxieties to the health worker.

   You are the health worker.   (Be your self as much as possible.) Your patient, a middle-aged male, has just been admitted to hospital following a blackout. You do not yet know the cause, and the patient remains unconscious. All vital signs are intact, but blood pressure is raised and there are signs of atypical reflexes on the patient's left side. The provisional diagnosis is one of cerebro-vascular accident (stroke). You cannot be sure until the patient has had a brain scan, or until they regain consciousness. The patient's relative has asked to see you.

2. *Situation:*   An out-patient / general practice clinic /occupational health department consultation for a chronic skin complaint. The patient has visited on four occasions with this complaint. There is no other significant medical history. However, the patient is a factory process worker producing electronic circuit

boards where he comes in to contact with chemicals. He lives and works in a depressed area with high unemployment.

Task: To deal with the patient's questions regarding their condition.

Time available: 5–10 minutes.

You are the patient. You are a factory worker making electronic circuit boards. The work is sometimes dirty, and you have to wear heavy protective clothing. The factory gets hot and stuffy in summer time. Over the last three months, you have developed a sharply defined skin rash over your trunk and left arm. It itches and is scaly. It is very uncomfortable especially when the temperature is hot. You have gone to see your health worker about this as you have been suffering from this condition now for three months. None of the creams you have been given has worked. Ask about the outcome of this. How long you will have it, what needs to be done to get better, etc.

You are the health worker. (Be yourself as much as possible.) The patient has psoriasis around his trunk and left arm, and has had it for three months. None of the standard treatments have had any effect. It is unlikely that the condition can be cured completely, though considerable relief might be obtained over a long period by use of combined drug and photic (ultra-violet light) therapy. There is essentially little that you can do for the patient. The condition may be aggravated by their working environment.

3. *Situation:* An occupational health worker has been admitted to an opthalmic ward following sudden onset visual disturbances in both eyes. The patient is on bed rest awaiting a visit from an opthalmic surgeon.

   Task: To deal constructively with the patient's questions.

   Time available: 5–10 minutes.

   You are the patient. (Be yourself as much as possible.) You work as an occupational health worker in a large commercial company office. You have two young children and are separated from your spouse. You have been admitted to hospital following a sudden deterioration of your eyesight. You have blurred eyesight with patchy loss of vision. You have been told you must rest on your back and can expect to have some treatment once the eye specialist has seen you. Your children are at present being looked after by your mother, but she is not in good health herself. You want to know what is wrong with you. Ask questions about your diagnosis and its implications; e.g. will you become blind?

You are the health worker. (Be yourself as much as possible.) Your patient has threatened detachment of the retina in both eyes. He is awaiting a visit from the opthalmic surgeon and some laser surgery may be necessary, but the extent of the problem is not yet known. The patient is not expected to lose his sight but may require strict horizontal bed rest for a period of time. If not, he may have complete retinal detachment and become blind.

Discussion

1. To what extent should the health worker be obliged to answer all the patient's questions, even when some may be unrealistic, such as to speculate on the effects of exotic or alternative treatments?

2. Who should be responsible for ensuring the patient's information needs are met, especially those involving difficult areas?

3. There are ethical dilemmas involved in the disclosure of information about sexual behaviour, abortion, under-age pregnancy, and so on, to a patient's relatives (husbands, wives, children). If you are asked direct questions about these areas by relatives, what might you do? Where does your responsibility to answer such questions begin and end?

4. Under what circumstances do you consider it acceptable not to answer patients' questions, and how might you go about responding when asked such questions in these circumstances?

5. Should parents always be consulted before answering a child's questions? Under what circumstances should this be done, and when not?

6. Do children have a right to honest answers to their questions from staff if their parents avoid giving such answers?

11

Breaking Bad News

Educational Objectives

By the end of this chapter , you should be able to

- recognize the effects of uncertainty on people under situations of high threat
- list reasons why health workers often avoid telling patients bad news
- list advantages and disadvantages of breaking bad news
- accept the appropriateness of patients being upset when given bad news
- recognize the right of patients to refuse treatment which may have uncertain benefits and considerable costs
- list the management advantages in disclosing bad news
- list the main responsibilities of the informer in regard to the breaking of bad news
- judge the appropriate timing for disclosure
- recognize the need to deal with feelings arising from the disclosure
- discuss the various common strategies used to avoid answering patient requests for disclosure
- recognize the important steps in planning for disclosure
- recognize the types of problem that may arise from intentions to protect the patient from bad news
- list the components of two or more strategies for breaking bad news
- carry out disclosure of bad news using both a sudden and gradual approach and provide effective follow-up

▦   Introduction

The necessity of bad news

Breaking bad news is something most health care professionals have to do, especially physicians and nurses. It can be difficult to do well. Health workers may be left feeling negative and critical of their skills. If this occurs too frequently health workers can become unhappy and demoralised. This leads to other problems.

There is a serious need to examine the disclosure of bad news for two reasons. First, we have already seen that information giving is often poor. This is particularly so when the information involves bad news (Blanchard, Labrecque, Ruckdescel and Blanchard, 1988; Gilhooly, Berkeley, McCann, Gibling and Murray, 1988, Fielding, Ko and Wong, 1995). Second, when it is carried out it is often done in a less than satisfactory way.

We cannot avoid the increasing demands by patients for information about their health status, especially when the situation is serious. However, while people react to bad news in different ways, the great majority feel worse when they face threat and uncertainty about what is going to happen to them. Research indicates that circumstances of concurrent high uncertainty and threat are among the most stressful and damaging that people can face.

There are many reasons for giving people bad news. This chapter explores why this should be done when there is a wish for such news (and why not when there is no such wish). It will also suggest how health workers might approach this difficult part of their role.

The right to know, or not

Few people enjoy giving bad news or upsetting or hurting others. The classical Greek kings must have agreed strongly with this, as they reputedly went so far as to kill messengers bearing bad news! We often delay or avoid giving bad news to others sometimes to the point of lying despite a belief that honesty is (usually) the best policy. Why is breaking bad news so difficult? Perhaps empathic understanding helps us anticipate how a person is going to feel when we give bad news. We know we wouldn't want to feel that way ourselves, thus we assume that putting someone else in that situation would cause similar reactions in them.

When we perceive ourselves contributing to the well-being of others, in a parental role, protectiveness may be increased. We may not adopt such roles willingly. Sometimes they evolve unnoticed in relationships with people who become dependent on us for certain things. We may collude, or collaborate unwittingly, to bring about with another person a relationship where we feel responsible for the emotional well-being of others, as parents may feel responsible for the well-being of their children.

These pressures are intensified where one perceives a professional responsibility for the physical well-being of a person, as health workers might do. When a poor outcome is anticipated, despite the best efforts of the health care team, a sense of failure or even guilt may be experienced. Then, not only is disclosure upsetting for the patient, it may also be perceived as an admission of failure by the health worker, causing self-doubt and blame.

Probably the most common reason for avoiding disclosure of bad news is that the health workers themselves become anxious. How do I disclose? How will the patients react? Will they get upset? Distressed? Hysterical? And then what will I do? How do I cope? What if they get sick, or have a cardiac arrest? What if they somehow are made worse by my act of disclosure? Better to not tell them; why upset them unnecessarily when it can't help to know? And anyway, they haven't asked.

It is not surprising that disclosure can provoke anxiety in health workers. Not only might the patient be upset, the unit manager or senior might not like it either. Add to this that most people don't like causing upset and there are some powerful reasons for avoiding disclosure.

Reasons for not disclosing bad news

Why should patients be told bad news if it will upset them, and if it is not going to alter the prognosis or worsen it? How important is disclosure anyway? To answer the second question first, disclosure seems to be very important. A number of studies have addressed the question of whether or not patients want bad news. These studies consistently report that the majority (92%) of patients want to know details of both diagnosis and prognosis, even when the news is bad (Blanchard et al, 1988). In many hospitals now, and in many general practice, nursing, and para-professional training programmes, informing patients is given a high priority. Despite the emphasis on disclosing bad news, it still seems to be carried out very inconsistently. A recent study in Scotland indicated that as many as one-third of patients with cancer died without having discussed their diagnosis with their general practitioners (Gilhooly et al, 1988), a situation little changed from that of 15 years earlier (Cartwright et al, 1973). In Hong Kong, the situation is no better (Fielding, Ko and Wong, 1995). More arguments are usually heard for not disclosing than for disclosing bad news.

Let's examine some of these arguments more closely. The major arguments can be divided into two main groups: not upsetting the patient, and loss of patient cooperation.

Don't upset the patient!

The first line of arguments for not disclosing bad news is based on the health workers' duty to keep patients happy and not to upest them. The patient may be unable to cope with the bad news, or the patient's condition may deteriorate.

The patient may commit suicide

While serious physical illness, particularly if HIV-related, is a risk factor for suicide (Rich et al, 1991; Gunnell and Frankel, 1994), there is little evidence to indicate that giving patients bad news increases risk of suicide (Hinton, 1972). 'Everybody knows someone' who had a patient who jumped out of a window, or who became hysterical and collapsed. Most reports of patients crumpling under the burden of bad news are anecdotal. When confirmed cases are examined more closely, many of the patients in question had pre-existing histories of difficulty in coping with crises. Again, such cases tend to be rare and have been explained as responses to the patient's sense of isolation or desire to avoid a painful or undignified experience. This more accurately reflects a lack of effective support for the patient than a hazard of disclosure (Hinton, 1972; Baile et al, 1993). Suicide risk is likely to be much reduced by providing effective counselling and support for patients and their families in stressful situations. Physician-assisted suicide (PAS) studies also indicate that organic mental disease, depression and personality issues are important variables in requests for PAS (Baile et al, 1993).

What such cases tell us is that careful evaluation of the patient before disclosure is important and that without it, over-disclosure can and does occur (see Chapter 9). What is much less apparent, because it seldom causes overt and sometimes dramatic reactions, is that under-disclosure is a far greater problem.

If patients are told bad news, they will deteriorate more rapidly

As for the argument that disclosure causes a patient's condition to deteriorate, the opposite again is likely to be the case. Most people begin to suspect that their condition is not good if they have progressive deterioration or if they become sick and don't get well again. In some cases patients may not yet suspect the seriousness of their diagnosis or prognosis. Where suspicions exist, so does uncertainty, and uncertainty is undesirable. Uncertainty generates feelings of anxiety — loss, suffering, or death — and these have physiological consequences which have marked effects on the body's ability to adapt. This is strongly suspected to impair healing processes, such as inflammatory responses and immunity (e.g. Ader, 1981). It may also cause demand crises in end organs, such as coronary vasospasm, leading to cardiac ischemia and increasing the risk of electrical disturbances, such as ventricular fibrillation (Rahe, 1989).

Less dramatic but no less important, uncertainty makes effective coping more difficult. It engenders feelings of helplessness, also associated with decreased survival (Seligman, 1975). Most people prefer the devil they know to the devil they don't know.

Patient cooperation suffers!

The second line of arguments against disclosure involves cooperation of the patient being in some way impaired by the disclosure. This interferes with health workers' ability to help the patient, and in this way the patient is harmed. These arguments can be subtle and persuasive but ultimately are reducible to one where the health workers retain control over patients. This is undesirable anywhere other than a police state.

The patient may refuse treatment

An extreme form of these arguments warns that patients, once told, become so uncooperative that they refuse treatment. This certainly does occur, but it is important to view this in context. Rejections of treatment are likely to occur most often when there appears to be poor prognosis and where the treatment offered may be perceived as painful or otherwise difficult to tolerate, and the expected benefits perceived to be small (Angell, 1984). Where such conditions exist, it is a reasonable choice to refuse aggressive attempts to slow down a disease process. This argument is often supplemented by the perceived risk of suicide if the patient is given bad news.

In conclusion, there appear to be few sustainable arguments for withholding bad news from people who want information on their health status. Bad news should not be given to patients only if they express a clear wish not to be told the nature of their circumstances. Such an expression may be verbal, non-verbal or both.

▆ Reasons why patients should be given bad news

Health workers must accept the responsibility of identifying the patients' information needs, of which bad news is but one aspect. In disclosing bad news, the process involves identifying patients' feelings. This requires sensitivity. It also needs commitment from the health worker to go through with disclosure and to be prepared to stay and provide support to the patient thereafter.

Uncertainty among health workers about how to handle expressions of emotion is a common reason for avoiding disclosure. Emotional expression is quite normal and should be acceptable, though many people are embarrassed when other people cry, for example. They may not feel confident about how to offer comfort, or may be tempted to try and achieve immediate comfort with unrealistic reassurance (see Chapters 9 and 10).

People do get upset when given bad news. Reactions to suffering are culturally influenced (Zbrowski, 1968; Littlewood, 1991) as well as being affected by personal style. Some cry quietly and withdraw, others are more flamboyant in their reactions, seeming almost hysterical, but virtually all people will show a reduction in their level of upset after a short time. Some people will not express feeling, reacting instead with numbed shock, or fear. All of these reactions are, for the most part, self-limiting and should not be feared by health workers. They will remain a source of embarrassment as long as the health worker is unfamiliar with handling emotion (see Chapter 8). It is a further responsibility of health workers who break bad news to provide room and time for people, at least initially, to adapt to the bad news they have been given. The majority of people, however, will probably not express florid emotion, keeping instead their feelings in check until they are alone.

Children are often not given bad news. Instead the parents are informed. Some health workers may then leave it to the parents to tell their children or not. This is inadequate for two reasons. First, it places an extreme burden on the parents who are struggling in most cases to cope with the implications of the news themselves. Second, the child may remain uncertain (but by no means ignorant) about their circumstances. This is particularly inadequate for adolescents, especially as patient participation in treatment maintenance is needed. Children have the right to be informed, just like everyone else (Alderson, 1993).

It is important to be sensitive to differences of culture. People with minority cultural backgrounds are often given less consideration as health care consumers. Uncertainty and anxiety characterize the communications between allopathic (Western) style health workers and other cultures.

Minority group members tend to have disproportionate levels of diagnoses such as schizophrenia (Littlewood and Lipsedge, 1989). They are also likely to have less access to information about their condition. With minority patients, special effort needs to be made to communicate on matters of bad news in a culturally sensitive manner.

Patient-protection and double-binds

A desire to protect the patient from bad news leads to a number of problems. Where the health worker is deciding whether to disclose bad news they may discuss the situation with a close relative, a parent, child or spouse first. The upset relative, trying to protect the patient, or for other reasons, requests the patient be not informed. The health worker may all too readily agree with this, thinking that the responsibility to disclose has been met and feeling relieved of an onerous task. However, the health worker must remember that, where the relative may provide helpful information on how the patient may be able to cope with the information, the health worker's first responsibility is towards the patient. Decisions regarding disclosure to the patient should be made on the basis of the patient's desires, not the relatives'.

Agreeing not to disclose bad news to a patient places all the health workers involved with that patient in a double-bind. If they do disclose, they may be accused by upset relatives. If they don't disclose they face being damned by an increasingly isolated and distressed patient. Under such circumstances effective care based on trust and respect becomes impossible. The strain of attempting to provide care under such conditions affects both patient, staff and thereby institutions in a highly negative way (see Chapter 13).

A special case: should children be given bad news?

In most cases where fatal illness is diagnosed, the parents will be the first to be told. This situation is perhaps one of the most difficult of all for parents to deal with. This represents a special case of withholding bad news. Most parents will find it very difficult to cope with the knowledge that their child is seriously ill and to discuss this with the child. The choice not to tell may be made primarily for these reasons. The parent's behaviour is often profoundly altered in relation to the family, resulting in a changed emotional climate.

The altered emotional climate of the home of a seriously ill child can generate considerable anxiety for the ill child and any siblings (Waechter,

1987). Parents may avoid discussion of the child's illness because they themselves cannot cope constructively with the implications. The child may be inhibited from expressing anxiety about the illness by the prevailing mood of the home, yet continue to experience high levels of anxiety which may not be recognized by parents. Parents may seriously underestimate the awareness of incurably ill children of their prognosis. Waechter (1987) identified 63% of a group of 16 fatally ill 6-to10-year-old children made comments related to loneliness, separation and death on a projective test (based on the Thematic Apperception Test). Only two of these children had been told their prognosis. Compared to three control groups of children with various non-fatal illness, reference to death was 'substantially more' (no numbers given) than among non-fatally ill children. Generalized anxiety was 'extremely high in all cases' of fatally ill children, being 'twice as high' as the scores of other hospitalized children.

An interesting finding of this study was a 'highly significant (positive) correlation between the total score on the projective test and the degree to which the child had been given an opportunity to discuss his fears and prognosis'. Waechter concluded. '. . . understanding, acceptance and conveyance of permission to discuss any aspect of his illness may decrease feelings of isolation, alienation, and the sense that his illness is too terrible to discuss completely'. A similar study of 20 leukemic children, however, found that 50% of mothers believed that the children (aged 6 to 10 years) should be told the 'whole truth', with 25% believing the child should be told the whole truth 'only when the child asks', and 25% believing the fatal nature of the prognosis should be withheld. Ten children were told of the possibility of death. This open communication extended to siblings, many of whom became involved in the patient's care (Krulik, 1987).

There is clearly a need for high levels of close support and counselling to be available to the family of a fatally ill child in order to help members deal with their feelings and to assist in supporting the adaptation of the family to a positive and healthy role in relation to the child. These issues are discussed more in Chapter 12.

Withholding bad news from children seems only to isolate them further from their needed support networks, as it does with adults. It should not be done unless the child expressly indicates a preference not to be told.

Staff protection

The disclosure of bad news is demanding of all persons involved, especially if the unit has a high proportion of seriously ill and vulnerable patients, e.g. child oncology units (Delvaux, Razavi and Farvacques, 1988). Thus, health workers employed in places where frequent disclosure of bad news is required could be prone to emotional burnout, and effective staff support is needed to prevent this. So, in addition to considerable responsibilities towards the patient, health workers, particularly those in managerial/supervisory roles, need to facilitate staff support. Further discussion of staff support can be found in Chapter 13. In addition, several other sources are available documenting counselling and support groups, frequent rotation and other strategies for minimizing staff burnout (e.g. Maguire and Faulkner, 1988).

Ethics and misinformation

Lies told to patients are seldom justifiable. Anecdotes of kindly GPs telling little old ladies who are dying that their complaint is 'not serious' (in order to spare them inevitable and purposeless worry) end with the old ladies living out their remaining days in blissful ignorance. Rarely will this have a place in the art of health care. There is a tremendous variety of situations in health settings where bad news needs to be given.

Should the health worker tell the truth, the whole truth and nothing but the truth, under all circumstances? Or is it acceptable to consider partial information, or even intentional misinformation, in order, say, to maintain hope in a patient? It has been stated that the patient's right to know the truth can be upheld while retaining room for hope (Cousins, 1979).

A key ethical point seems to be the health worker's responsibility to the patient. In meeting that responsibility, the health worker is obliged first to avoid harming the patient in any way, thereafter, to minimize any suffering, and then to do whatever possible to restore the patient to health. If restoration of health is not possible, limiting further deterioration assumes a substitute priority. Minimizing suffering is always an obligation. As chronic, non-life-threatening diseases become the dominant health problems, quality of life becomes a greater issue. In failing to disclose information to a patient, bad as well as good, the patient is deprived of the opportunity to make informed decisions about how to live their remaining life. Providing information permits patients both to accept greater responsibility for, and control over, their health and life, and to make decisions about their future care. Withholding information removes both control and responsibility from the patient who may suffer more. Thus it is hard to see how the patient's interests are being served by withholding information.

When, where, and with whom?

Under what circumstances is disclosure desirable? When is the best time? Should it be done in the privacy of a room, or on the open ward? Should the patient be alone with the doctor, or, should relatives or other staff be present?

When?

Where possible patients should be given information at the time they request it, even though the staff may not think it either optimal or desirable. There are important reasons for this. Patients make requests for information because they want to know. The phrasing of the question and the patients' general manner are additional information for the health worker. People who ask for information become very frustrated when they are not provided with clear and succinct answers. The timing may seem highly inappropriate to the staff, but patients often feel differently. Consider the following example of a woman who was given cardiopulmonary resuscitation for a cardiac arrest in a casualty department:

> After it happened I was terrified. I mean nobody could calm me. I knew something had happened that shouldn't have happened, and I was absolutely terrified. And no one could calm me, everyone was saying 'Calm down, calm down' and I'm saying 'What's happening, what's going on', you know, it was a real . . . , *but I needed to know what had happened* 'cos it was so strong. 'You have to tell me', you know, they're saying 'Breathe through your nose', 'No, tell me what happened', and I kept thinking, I'm sure I've had a heart attack, but no one's going to say it to me.

Here in the aftermath of a medical emergency, the patient is expected to lie back and do she was told, without questioning or expecting information. For some patients, this may be possible, but for many it is too much to ask. Could the staff say anything to the patient under such circumstances, without precipitating cardiac arrest?

What can you think of saying that would have been appropriate? There was a lot that could be said; 'You passed out and we're trying to make sure everything is OK'; 'Your heart was beating irregularly, which made you pass out, but we have steadied it. We need your help now. Please breathe through your nose', and so forth would have served to inform the patient without causing unnecessary terror.

Even though saving the patient's life is a priority in this example, patient cooperation would likely have been facilitated by telling the patient her circumstances. Even if the patient was upset by the news, the physiological effect and lack of cooperation would probably be no greater than that from the patient's anxiety about what had happened, and may be less. Using ADA is not always appropriate or possible. There may be no time to assess need, but it is reasonable to assume that the patient, in asking, expresses a need. When this happens, staff should have the confidence and support of colleagues to answer honestly.

Under less urgent circumstances, when patients ask for information that requires disclosure of bad news, it may indicate that there has been insufficient information given, or that the staff have not approached the patients to discuss with them their condition. It is important that constant communication is maintained between medical, nursing and other staff and patients regarding their conditions, under all circumstances. There is no justification for not doing so. When constant communication is maintained, patients are better informed and thus in a better position to contribute to decision making regarding their management. Also more frequent and easier situations exist for the disclosure of bad news, as and when necessary.

Where a patient asks a difficult question of a health worker, it is indefensible as an avoidance strategy to say:

I don't know, I'll get someone to come and tell you.

Rushing to consult with others should not be done at this time. Management decisions regarding disclosure need to be made before, or at the latest, at the same time that information becomes available, as with other aspects of patient care. Preferably, they should occur before the patient is admitted if hospitalized. This requires a pre-existing policy for staff to disclose any bad news if/when the patient requests information, and not to decide only 'if the situation arises'. Any delay may be very telling to the patient, increasing uncertainty and decreasing trust if questions evoke: 'I'll get someone else'. By keeping patients informed of developments in their case, these situations should not arise.

The kind of situations where very junior staff are confronted with serious 'bad news' questions are themselves illuminating. Where good communications exist between staff and patients, they will rarely arise. On the other hand, their frequent occurrence suggests that generally communications policy between staff and patients may benefit from a review.

> ### *Key Points*
>
> Planning information management is just as important as plan-
> ning other aspects of patient management. Decisions on disclosure
> need to be made **in anticipation** of the disclosure, not after re-
> quests for information have begun.
>
> Avoid 'accumulation' of bad news by keeping patients informed
> of their condition and the implications of their test results and
> treatment, as the information becomes available.
>
> Use an ADA model (Assessment, Disclosure, Assimilation; Chap-
> ter 9) to develop unit policy.

Where?

This is quite straightforward. Bad news should be disclosed in private,
where the patient is able to discuss the implications of the news with the
health worker. Hospital corridors, crowded and busy wards, and the presence of a group of students and other people are strictly inappropriate. To
tell patients during a ward round that they have untreatable cancer, for
example, indicates lack of sensitivity and sheer ignorance of the implications of such news for the patients. Patients given information under such
circumstances are discounted as no more than a vehicle for a disease. If
the patient asks the question during a ward round, it may need to be dealt
with then. In so doing, the person in charge should give the news in as
sensitive a manner as possible. But that these questions must be asked at
ward rounds implies that patient access to informed staff is inadequate.

Ideally, a room should be available where there can be some privacy
and where the individuals should not be disturbed either by others entering or leaving, even if it means moving to a different part of the hospital
or clinic to find such a room. Every health care facility should have
available one room for this purpose. Outside hospital, a private room in a
health centre, or even in the patient's own home is adequate. If necessary
find a quiet park bench.

Curtains shield eyes but not ears and provide inadequate privacy to
disclosure events. Nonetheless, some patients are not able to move in a
wheelchair or alone to the privacy of a room. It may be necessary to
consider deferring disclosure until privacy can be obtained, perhaps by
moving the bed. Sometimes, this will not be possible. An elderly patient
on ICU who is partially deaf may be difficult to talk with privately.

Staff should, as a team, attempt to identify possible solutions to these more difficult disclosure situations by effective planning to anticipate their occurrence. Strategies might be identifiable for overcoming many of the difficulties. Some situations will be less than perfect. In cases where no solution is available, staff need to decide case by case whether disclosure or privacy is more important to the patient.

With whom?

As with other areas of communication, there are no absolute fixed rules about who discloses, and who else is present. Probably no more that two health workers, the patient and one close relative, such as the spouse, or the parents of a child would be a natural group for such an exercise. One health worker and the patient or relative is often the norm. This may vary to suit cultural needs. The presence of a close relative provides support for the patient when substantial bad news is disclosed, and informs the relative simultaneously. (Bear in mind the patient may have the additional burden of coping with a distraught relative.)

Again, by discussing these issues at first contact, along with other demographic information gathering, many of these difficulties can be avoided.

Who discloses the information? French (1979) reported patients preferred technical, diagnostic and prognostic information from doctors, while nurses were preferred for morale-building information. However, in the years since this study was carried out, nurses' roles as information providers put them in a good position to disclose. Disclosure of bad news may occur in community settings, and it may be up to a health visitor to discuss the implications of some information.

The increasing inclusion of communication skills programmes within professional training courses, should produce a wider range of people able to give patients the information they desire.

However, if the health worker feels unsure of being able to deal with the patient's technical questions, or if decisions need to be made regarding treatment options, then the doctor may be the most appropriate person to disclose the news. Also, the doctor should be sufficiently confident about dealing effectively with the range of questions a patient may ask. Similarly, a doctor may be unable to answer a patient's questions about a treatment course of, for example radiotherapy, and may ask a radiotherapist to deal with this.

One final matter is that bad news may increase the patients' level of arousal so much that they cannot take in the information that is given to them. Though they may be able to discuss the issue at the time, they may have little recall of the information after the event. Returning to see the patient after a short time gives the patient opportunities for clarification. Some hospital units provide written information, or tape recordings of information for patients following certain events, such as acute myocardial infarction. Patient recall of information is notoriously poor, even under good conditions. When patients are highly aroused, anxious or distraught following bad news, they may need information supplements later. (See also Chapter 9.)

Preparation and ADA

The disclosure of bad news can be considered to have three phases:
1. Assessment
2. Disclosure
3. Assimilation

The term ADA refers to these three phases.

Assessment

Assessment of information needs has been covered in Chapter 9. Only a brief discussion and some examples are therefore presented here.

Blanket disclosure of bad news to every one is undesirable. Different people want, or can cope with different levels of information about their situation. Some form of preparatory assessment of the patient's information needs before disclosing bad news is therefore mandatory if appropriate levels of information are to be given.

How do you tell whether the patient wants to know the bad news?. There are several ways to find out. The best way is to ask patients if they want themselves, or someone nominated on their behalf, to be kept informed. This can be done as part of the admission interview or the provisional patient assessment. Then it is unobtrusive and straightforward.

After identifying the patient's desire to be kept informed, it is important to identify the patient's immediate needs for information.

You may have to be prepared to spend some time talking with the patient to achieve this. There is no substitute for this, other than if the patient requests information by a direct question, and even then some preparation is appropriate.

Key Points

The routine assessment of patients' information needs and desires is currently carried out in many types of practice. There are areas of practice where this information is not *routinely* gathered. Should a decision need to be made on disclosing bad news to a patient, the lack of data on the patient's information preferences makes finding out more difficult this time.

Therefore routine collection of this information on admission to hospital or enrolment into a clinic, or on first contact along with name, address and birth date is strongly recommended as a policy (see Chapter 9).

The following exchange illustrates the kind of approach that might be taken in an exploratory discussion to evaluate a person's desire for information.

HW: Good morning Mrs Kay, how are you feeling today?

Pt: Oh, I'm all right. A bit tired.

HW: My name is Pat Lee, one of your nurses. We met yesterday, do you remember?

Pt: Yes, yes . . . ah, . . . hello.

HW: You said you were feeling a bit tired. Did you have trouble sleeping last night?

Pt: Well, it was a bit noisy and my chest was . . . uncomfortable, but they, ah, gave me something to help, ah . . . make me sleep. But I feel today quite weary, you know, . . . weak.

HW: How do you feel about that?

Pt: Oh, well . . . ah . . . I've . . . ah . . . I wish I could feel more lively, but I don't seem to have any energy anymore.

HW: Has any one explained why you might be feeling weak and tired?

Pt: No. No one.

HW: What do you think is the reason for your feeling tired?

Pt: Well . . . .ah . . . I suppose . . . my illness, but I thought . . . I'd be, you know, feeling better by now. After my last attack . . . I just haven't had any energy. It . . . ah . . . it takes me all my time to, to just lie here.

HW: Is it a worry for you?

Pt: Yes! . . . I'm usually . . . , I usually have lots of energy, rushing around all the time . . . I thought I . . . it's been nearly a week, is it, since I first came in here?

HW: Go on.

Pt: I just didn't expect . . . didn't think I'd have another . . . ah . . . attack, an' . . . ah . . . y'know . . . what with the jumping on my chest, and . . . the pain . . . oh, it was terrible! I don't want to go through that again, . . . no, . . . so . . .

HW: It must have been very scary for you.

Pt: Oh, . . . yes, it was, it was. I am scared, ... I don't want . . . ah . . . . we've all got to die, I know that. I don't want to die, but wishing won't stop it, . . . ah . . . so, . . . ah . . . I don't know, I don't know . . . .

HW: You said no one talked to you about your illness recently?

Pt: Ah . . . no, no. They . . . ah, the doctor . . . said, . . . told me they had to . . . ah . . . that my heart stopped . . . and they restarted it. But I just keep feeling . . .

HW: Feeling what?

Pt: Oh that, . . . the . . . ah . . . heart's not in such good . . . ah . . . shape.

HW: Would you like to talk about that?

Pt: Well, . . . yeah, I . . . want to know what's . . . going on . . . yes.

This exchange now leads naturally and comfortably into a discussion of the patient's condition. The health worker, both by empathic understanding and sensitivity to the patient's verbal and non-verbal cues, picked up the likely anxiety the patient was experiencing about her condition. Most people in these circumstances are probably experiencing some degree of appropriate anxiety. This may not be overt and they may appear almost unconcerned about their illness. This is one way of coping with the inherent feelings. Coping with anxiety may make some people more alert for clues about their situation, while others may become blunted to their surroundings, preferring instead not to be interested in what is happening (Miller, 1987). Probing may not reveal anxiety, and an accompanying avoidance or unwillingness to discuss the illness suggests the patient is coping by avoiding confrontation with the implications of their illness. Then it is inappropriate to push information. Rarely is it necessary to do so.

Bear in mind that many patients are depressed but that depressive signs are frequently missed in hospitalized patients, particularly if the patient is in pain (Maguire, 1984b).

Key Points

Before giving information, find out what and how much information patients already know about their situation. This may require you to confirm suspicions already held by the patient.

Use of empathic understanding may help to identify an 'entry' to discuss the patient's information needs.

Disclosure

Having identified the patient's desire for information, the second phase of ADA involves disclosing the bad news to the patient.

All too often for in-patients, information is disclosed at the bedside by health workers looking down on the patient during a ward round. It may be given to the relatives in a hospital corridor, as happens in 25% of coronary care units in New Zealand (Holdaway, 1985). These practices are really very poor. It is seldom helpful to say:

> If you have any questions, ask one of the staff and we'll send someone for a chat.

Remarks like these are vague and impersonal and tend to trivialize the patient's concerns. Then the ward round moves on to the next bed and the patient is left in a state of shock trying to figure things out. In New Zealand, only 21% of relatives of dying patients in coronary care units had any kind of follow up from the hospital (Holdaway, 1985). In the case of an out-patient, it is not sufficient to spend only five minutes discussing bad news before pushing the patient out and seeing the next one.

Basic preparation is needed before disclosure. When the health worker knows in advance that the patient will probably be given some information, preparation could include some or all of the following:
- arrange for a close relative to be available
- familiarize oneself with the details of the case
- prepare material to enable estimates to be made of prognostic likelihoods
- discuss with colleagues about cross-referral for special treatments (e.g. radiotherapy, etc.)
- tell the patient/relative that you would like to discuss results, etc. with the family/ parent/child

It is possible to prepare in this way when the patient asks a question spontaneously. Again, if the information is available, it should be disclosed at this time. It is inappropriate to defer the disclosure until 'all the results are in' (unless they are confirmatory of a diagnosis), or until 'I've had chance to discuss it with my colleagues'. That may need to happen later. Given the definition of bad news as being of substantial impact on a patient's life, the health worker should consider several meetings to fully provide the information and help assimilate the news. Therefore, meetings with colleagues can take place later, the information from these being given in a subsequent meeting with the patient.

Assimilation

Thus, some time needs to be spent with the patient after the bad news has been broken to help the patient come to terms with the information. The news may be disclosed in stages or it may be disclosed all at once. With either approach, the health worker must be prepared to meet with the patient on two or three occasions to clarify that assimilation has occurred and the patient is coping effectively.

In Chapter 3, it was argued that coping with bad news involves a process of adapting to an altered framework of self-world reference. The process seems to entail a gradual self-desensitization to the fearful nature of the threat, what patients describe as making sense of the event, or in this case information, in terms of their life experience (Thorne, 1993).

Though this assimilation often takes place naturally, it can be very disruptive to the patients and their families. As adaptation proceeds, further questions will occur, extra information or confirmation will be needed by the patients and their families. The health worker must therefore be personally available to answer additional questions. If this is not possible, another person (acceptable to the patient and family) should be identified early to fulfil that role.

This is a time for staff to place priority on the psychosocial needs of the patient. This does not mean automatically calling for a psychiatrist, psychologist or even social worker. Rather, the staff need to make themselves available to talk, to spend time with the patient, answer questions or hold hands. This is particularly important when the patient has no family or is otherwise unsupported. There may be circumstances when the staff must try to fill the gap left by the absence of the patient's family, for example AIDS patients may be rejected by their families. Families of children with serious illness also need close support. This can undoubtedly be difficult but is a highly important aspect of patient care.

Where the news is not life-threatening and adaptation to living with the disease is important for effective management (e.g. diabetes), it is imperative to provide psychosocial care of the nature described. Jacobson and colleagues (Jacobson et al, 1990) identified three variables present at diagnosis which predicted adherence to three aspects of treatment (insulin, diet and monitoring) four years later in a group of adolescent diabetics. These variables were adaptive strength, 'ego-strength' , and locus of control, all of which reflect elements of control over coping ability. Age was also an important influence with pre-adolescents adapting better than adolescents. Others have identified similar effects (Laron, 1989).

Thus, assessment of how well the patients are adjusting to their changed circumstance (or bad news) has a significant role to play in effective care delivery.

Technique

There are probably two main approaches to disclosing bad news. 'Sudden disclosure (strategies B and D below), and the stepwise or gradual disclosure approach (strategies A and C below). Both approaches have advantages and disadvantages. There is no one right way, though the stepwise approach is often favoured because it offers greater control over the extent of disclosure. In contrast, the full disclosure approach offers the advantage of dealing with the full implications at one sitting (strategy D easier, strategy B more difficult). Use the technique that you feel most comfortable with. Indeed, it is recommended, as with all other techniques in this book, that students develop their own style of practice, using the described methods as starting points. Let's examine both strategies in turn.

Strategies for disclosing bad news can be classified into four types:

		Rate of disclosure	
		Gradual	Sudden
Amount	Partial	A	B
disclosed	Total	C	D

The full disclosure approach

As the title suggests, this strategy involves disclosing the full nature of the bad news at one go, then spending time helping the patient come to terms with the information. This requires commitment, for once begun, there is no turning back and the health worker must be prepared to spend time not only in answering any questions, but also in helping the recipient to adjust to the information afterwards.

HW: Good afternoon, Mr White, I wonder if I might have a word with you? You may remember me, my name is Kay, I work with Dr Lee your consultant.

Pt: Afternoon, yes?

HW: How are you feeling today?

Pt: Oh, pretty much the same, y'know, very tired.

HW: Tired?

Pt: Yeah, all the time, an' it can't be because I'm not getting enough rest, haha.

HW: Why do *you* think you're feeling so tired?

Pt: Well, I suppose it's me illness, I, ah, oh I don't seem to have any strength . . .

HW: Is that worrying you?

Pt: If it isn't the 'flu, then it must be pretty serious.

HW: Hmm, I'm afraid it is.

Pt: Oh God, I knew it.

(Health worker waits for patient to respond.)

Pt: Is it cancer?

HW: What makes you think of cancer?

Pt: My Father died of cancer and he just dried up and got weaker and weaker. He was as strong as an ox. It seems like I'm going the same way. Is it cancer?

HW: Well, yes, you're right, it is cancer. As you know, we did some tests on you yesterday, and we've got the results, and . . .

Pt: Oh . . . (pause). Are you sure?

HW: Yes, there no doubt about it, I'm sorry to say.

(Long pause — health worker waits for patient to digest this information before going on.)

Pt: Can, . . . is there anything you, . . . is it treatable, or . . . what?

HW: Well, there are certainly treatments we can . . . give you to help control it, but I'm afraid it has spread a bit now and that limits the kind of treatments that we can use.

(Pause.)

HW: One of the things we need to talk about in the next day or so are the options for treatment.

Pt: You can treat it, then?

HW: That's what we need to discuss.

(Pause; patient does not pursue discussion of treatment.)

HW: Did you suspect that it was cancer you had?

Pt: Er..weell, you know, I felt so well before I started to lose weight and I thought it was probably..something. As I said, the same thing happened to my father, see . . . he, er . . . he had er cancer.

HW: This must be quite a shock to you.

Pt: Yeah, you never . . . , y'know . . . , it seems an impossible thing to happen to you; it happens to everyone else but it seems impossible to happen to you, hahaha, (sigh).

Pt: What . . . how much, how much can, er, you do? I mean.

HW: That depends to an extent on what you want. First, we will make sure that you're kept comfortable and free of discomfort. In addition, we can put you on a course of drugs to shrink the tumours which in some cases keeps it under control for quite a long time. Some people find that unpleasant, but others tolerate it quite well. We wouldn't know how you would react to the drugs 'til we tried them. There aren't really any other approaches we can use just now.

Pt: What about radiation?

HW: If the tumour has spread to several sites, it is very difficult to treat with radiotherapy, or surgery. Those approaches are really only suitable where there are only one or two tumours.

Pt: How many have I got then?

HW: In your case there are more.

Pt: How many more?

HW: We're not sure. We know of three, and there are probably some smaller sites we haven't found yet.

Pt: Three! . . .

Pt: What, . . . ah, how long will it be if I didn't have the drug treatment?

HW: It's very difficult to say for any individual. What we can say is that only about 40% of people with your type and stage of cancer are alive after six months without drugs. With drugs, we can get better than 60% survival for six months, about 20% of people a lot longer.

There is one thing to bear in mind, and that is that a very small percentage of people with quite advanced cancer do show quite remarkable improvement, sometimes complete recovery. We don't know why this happens. In addition, there are quite a few things you could do to help maintain your health. We can discuss these later, if you like.

Pt: Oh, I don't think I can cope with this . . . its, its all a bit much to take in right now. I had no idea, I thought it would be, like years or something . . .

HW: It's a very scary thing to have to face.

Pt: Yeah, very. (eyes begin to water).

(Long pause.)

HW: I expect you're feeling very confused right now, hmmm?

Pt: Yeah. I was thinking about life and death this morning, y'know, what brought it on was looking at the death columns in the paper, thinking it could have been me there today, and thinking wonder why he died, y'know? But I never really thought . . . Phew. I'm glad you told me though. I'd rather know, I need to find out as much as I can about it.

HW: If you want to know anything else, ask for me.

(Pause.)

HW: Is your wife coming to visit you this afternoon?

Pt: Er, yes . . . . . Don't know how she'll take it.

HW: Is that a worry for you?

Pt: Yes, I don't think she had thought it was that serious.

HW: I haven't spoken to your wife yet. If you like I could see the two of you later, or I could ask our nurse counsellor to come and talk with you. Whichever way, I'll come and see you again later. Would you like me to tell your wife?

Pt: No, I think . . . I think I'd better tell her. Maybe we could talk to the nurse?

HW: I'll arrange that, and if you have any questions for me, then write them down because people often forget them when it comes to discussions. Is there anything we can do for you right now?

Pt: No, no thanks, I think I need to, y'know, think about it a bit.

The above exchange is a composite that serves to illustrate several features of the full-disclosure and mop-up approach:

• The health worker made some, albeit cursory evaluation of the patient's readiness to receive information by asking: 'Why do you think you're feeling so tired'. This lead to the patient raising the issue of cancer.

- The health worker used a reflective question form to clarify the nature of the patient's suspicion 'Why do you think of cancer?', revealing the patient's suspicion that he had this disease.

- Note how the health worker quickly got to the full disclosure of the true nature of the patient's condition. The worst points of the news were presented in the earliest stages of the (shortened) discussion.

- When the patient asks 'How long?' the health worker wisely avoids giving a precise estimation (which is usually impossible anyway), whilst balancing the benefits and costs of chemotherapy in a fair manner, and giving room to participate in the treatment decision, if desired.

- The health worker maintains room for realistic hope by indicating that some small percentage of patients do survive much longer than others, even into complete remission.

- The health worker makes some attempt to assess the patient's emotional reaction to the news, offering further counselling if desired.

- The health worker avoids the use of false or inappropriate reassurance. The patient's condition is obviously serious; to pretend otherwise would be very misleading.

On the negative side, there was little exploration of the patient's willingness to receive, or abilities to cope with the full extent and implication of the diagnosis and prognosis. Similarly, little subsequent discussion was offered by the health worker, and delving into the patient's ability to cope with the news was scanty. Information was presented in an unstructured way; the health worker's attempts at encouraging hope were largely unheard by the patient. Nonetheless, the exchange serves to illustrate the strategy of sudden disclosure.

The step-wise approach

This style of disclosure allows periodic evaluation of patients' information needs and coping ability, permitting finer control over the amount and type of information disclosed. It also increases the patients' control by allowing them to stop disclosure if they feel too threatened. However, when information is released in stages, sensitivity is required to help the patient adapt to each stage. In short this approach probably requires a greater degree of rapport and empathy with the patient than does the previous approach. The following example, again a composite, illustrates the same case dealt with using the gradual disclosure approach.

HW: Good afternoon, Mr White, I wonder if I might have a word with you? You may remember me, my name is Kay, I work with Dr Lee, your consultant.

Pt: Afternoon, yes?

HW: How are you feeling today?

Pt: Oh, pretty much the same, y'know, very tired.

HW: Tired?

Pt: Yeah, all the time, an' it can't be because I'm not getting enough rest, haha.

HW: Why do *you* think you're feeling so tired?

Pt: Well, I suppose it's me illness, I, ah . . . if it's not the 'flu then it must be pretty serious to make me feel like this.

HW: What makes you say that?

Pt: Well, I'm not feeling any better. It's been three weeks now, and I've lost almost six kilos of weight in the last three months. That's a lot.

HW: Yes, it is. What do you think is wrong with you?

Pt: Well, I don't know. That's what I'm in here to find out, hahaha.

HW: Has anyone suggested anything, or do you have any thoughts about it?

Pt: Well, no, and I mean it's not right to feel like this is it? I had some tests done earlier in the week but they've not had the results back yet, so . . .

HW: Well, that's right, we did some tests on you yesterday, and we've got the results now.

Pt: Oh, am I all right, or . . . what?

HW: I'm afraid things don't look as good as we'd hoped.

Pt: Oh . . . .what's up? Is it serious?

HW: Yes, I'm afraid it looks like it might be.

(Patient looks expectantly at health worker.)

HW: Would you like to know the results?

Pt: Yes, tell me, please.

HW: Well, the X-rays we did earlier this week showed a slight shadow, and when we had a look inside your lung yesterday we found a lump.

Pt: A lump?

HW: Yes.

(Pause.)

HW: Had it occurred to you that there might be a problem with your chest?

Pt: No, I . . . er, what kind of lump?

HW: Well, when we looked at it yesterday we found it to be a bit . . . ah, difficult to get at.

Pt: Is it serious? Can you treat it?

HW: I think it is quite serious, yes. It does need to be dealt with soon in some way as it will become a problem.

(Pause.)

HW: Would you like to know more?

Pt: There's more?, . . . oh God!

HW: Would you like to think about what I've said so far and talk about it some more later?

Pt: I've got cancer, haven't I?

HW: What makes you think of cancer?

Pt: My father died of cancer and he just dried up and got weaker and weaker. He was as strong as an ox. It seems like I'm going the same way. Is it cancer?

HW: We think it might be, yes.

Pt: Oh . . . . ha, I had a feeling . . .

HW: (pause) A feeling about what?

Pt: That it might be cancer.

HW: It seems it's still quite a shock to you.

Pt: Yeah. (pause) You never . . . , y'know . . . , it seems an impossible thing to happen to you; it happens to everyone else but it seems impossible to happen to you, hahaha, (sigh). What . . . how much, how much can, er, you do? I mean, how serious is it?

HW: Well, we're rather limited in the treatments we can use. Because of where the lump is, it's quite closely involved with some other structures in the chest, and that means we can't do surgery.

Pt: You said there was more . . .

HW: Er, (sigh) yes. We thought there were some aspects of your illness we couldn't put down to a lung problem, your backache for example, so when we did the scans yesterday we looked at other places.

Pt: . . . and?

HW: That showed some . . . other lumps.

Pt: Oh . . . God! How many? Where?

HW: There are three that we know of.

Pt: Where?

HW: One in your left lung and two in your lower back.

Pt: Three! Are they all . . . ?

HW: We think they are tumours.

Pt: Phew . . . what can you do? Will I have to have radium treatment?

HW: Well, we need to discuss the treatment options available. There are three points to make. First, it's important to bear in mind that we will make sure that you're kept as comfortable as possible. Remember that. Second, we can put you on a course of chemotherapy, drugs to shrink the tumours which will probably keep it under control for some time. Some people find the drug therapy very unpleasant, but others tolerate it quite well. We wouldn't know how you would react to the drugs 'til we tried them. Third, there are quite a few things you could do to help maintain your health. We can talk about that in more detail later if you like.

Pt: What about radiation?

HW: Because the tumour has spread to several sites, it is very difficult to treat with radiotherapy, or surgery. Radiotherapy will help to keep the tumour in your lung in check. As a curative approach, it's really only suitable where there is only one tumour site. In your case there are several.

Pt: What, . . . ah, what would happen if I didn't have the drug treatment?

HW: It's very difficult to say for any individual. What we can say is that about 40% of people with your type and stage of cancer are alive after six months without drugs. With drugs, we can get better than 60% survival for six months, about 20% of people a lot longer. Some people a long time.

Pt: Only six months . . .

(Pause.)

Pt: It's funny, I was thinking about life and death this morning, y'know, what brought it on was looking at the death columns in the paper, thinking It could have been me there today, and thinking wonder why he died, y'know? But I never really thought . . . Phew.

HW: It's a difficult thing to face. Is your wife coming to visit you this afternoon?

Pt: Er, yes, ...don't know how she'll . . . take it.

HW: Is that a worry for you?

Pt: Yes, I don't think she had thought it was that serious.

HW: I haven't spoken to your wife yet. If you like I could see the two of you later, or I could ask our nurse counsellor to come and talk with you. Whichever way, I'll come and see you again later. Would you like me to tell your wife?

Pt: No, I think I'd better tell her. Maybe we could talk to the nurse?

HW: I'll arrange that, and if you have any questions for me, then write them down because people often forget them when it comes to discussions. Is there anything we can do for you right now?

Pt: No, no thanks, I think I need to, y'know, think about it a bit.

HW: I would like to tell you something. A very small percentage of people with quite advanced cancer do show quite remarkable improvement, sometimes complete recovery. We don't know why this happens. So it's important to retain hope.

Pt: Yes, . . . thanks.

This composite example illustrates the main features of the step-wise or gradual disclosure method.

- The health worker more carefully assesses the patient's perceptions of the illness to both evaluate the patient's information needs and as an introduction to the disclosure.
- The health worker again uses the reflective question to evaluate the patient's thoughts about the condition.
- The disclosure of the first 'unit' of the bad news is quite gentle, that the test results show 'things don't look as good as we'd hoped', leaving the patient to indicate desire for more information, or unwillingness to know more.
- The patient responds with a question which the health worker answers precisely: 'Is it serious?' 'Yes, I'm afraid it looks like it is'. Note the use of ' . . . I'm afraid . . . ' which indicates both gravity and concern. This further indicates the seriousness of the patient's condition. It acts both as a lure or a warning to the patient. The patient can then choose to ask for more or end the disclosure at that point.
- When the lump is mentioned, the health worker moves away from further disclosure to ask if the patient had considered a chest complaint to be a possibility. This gives the patient a chance to move away from discussing the increasingly threatening nature of the conversation.
- Again, the use of 'ah, difficult to get at', is purposefully ambiguous. Some patients will want clarification of the meaning, but for others it is 'precise' enough at this stage in the disclosure.
- When the health worker asks if the patient wants to know more, the health worker has sensed that the patient is beginning to be a bit overwhelmed with the implications of the news and is offering to stop, while signalling there is more.

- When the patient raises the issue of cancer, the health worker tentatively says 'we think so', rather than 'yes'. This allows the health worker to move slowly here since the patient's reactions to this very threatening diagnosis is not certain.
- Later the patient picks up the issue of 'more bad news', indicating a desire to know more. This leads to disclosure of metastatic disease, and then into a preliminary discussion of treatment options.

The step-wise approach offers a much more gradual build up of the bad news, allowing the health worker to control news if the patient seems to be having difficulty coping. Remember it is quite appropriate for people to be shocked and upset by news such as the examples provide, and this in itself is not a reason to terminate the disclosure. Only if the recipient appears to be having difficulty coping with news, requests no further information, or requests a chance to consider what has already been disclosed, should the disclosure be temporarily halted.

Key Points

If unsure whether to continue, simply ask the patient if more information is required.

Disclosure with children

Considering disclosing bad news to children can be daunting. There is an expectation that an elderly adult has had 'a good life' and will get sick. But for children whose lives have 'just begun', it is considered tragic when debilitating sickness occurs. This is particularly true with severe chronic, or terminal disease such as cancer.

However, by removing much of the uncertainty the child's task is eased. Ask the children on admission if they want to be involved in their care. While children are more vulnerable to the stress generated by uncertainty than adults, they are often more adaptable than adults. They have more naive concepts of illness and death (see Chapter 3). This can influence their understanding and acceptance of information. Older children, especially adolescents present a greater coping challenge. Adolescents understand the implications of illness and death and may feel cheated of life in a way a younger child does not. Younger children may fail to fully comprehend the seriousness of a diagnosis, but often can understand that parental distress signals something serious.

Disclosure to children should be done by a member of staff with whom the patient has a good and trusting relationship. The parent(s) should be present when the discussion occurs. Below is one example of how such a disclosure might occur.

(After establishing rapport with the patient.)

HW: Kevin, we think we know why you have been ill. Would you like me to tell you what's wrong?

Pt: Am I ill?

HW: Yes, you are. Would you like me to explain what's happened?

Pt: (Nods.)

HW: When your body makes new blood, which it does all the time, it takes a while to do so properly. We don't know why, but sometimes a body makes too much new blood too quickly.

(Pause.)

Pt: Have I got too much new blood?

HW: You have too much new blood.

HW: Your blood is OK in other ways. But it can't stop germs from hurting you and that means you can get very sick because the germs can take over. It's hard for us to stop germs from hurting you.

Pt: Will I have to have some medicine?

HW: We can give you medicine to help stop the germs this time. It's harder for us to get your blood to do it. We are also helping your blood and giving you some more blood in these bags.

Pt: Am I going to die?

HW: No, we don't think so. We think we can make you better again. But we will have to give you some very strong medicine to do that. If we don't give you the medicine, then you could.

(Pause.)

Pt: Will I have to have an injection?

HW: Yes, several. Sometimes the medicine can make you feel quite ill. But it makes most children better after a while.

(Pause.)

Mother: Mummy, Daddy, Susan and other doctors and nurses in the hospital are going to do their best to make you well again.

HW: Are you worried about the injections.

Pt: (Nods.)

HW: It's hard to be ill like this. Would you like to meet some other children who had the medicine and are getting better now? They can tell you about it, then you, your Mum and Dad and I can help you decide what you want to do. Does that sound all right?

Pt: Yes.

HW: Good. If you want to ask me anything at all, you can, OK?

The health worker has tried to explain conceptually to the child the type of problem causing the illness. Kevin is just five years old. At this age, death may still be understood as a reversible event. As such it may not be as threatening to the child as the prospect of injections. In an older child of six years or more, death is viewed as an irreversible event, but one that is capricious and distant to the child. What is threatening is the possibility of separation for the child.

Foley and McCarty (1976) describe a 'typical physician's explanation to a leukemic child of school age':

> You have a serious blood disease, leukemia. Ten years ago, there was no treatment for leukemia and many people died. Now there are a number of drugs which can be used to treat leukemia. There are several types of leukemia and the type you have in the one for which there are the most drugs. Treatment to keep the leukemia cells away will last three years. You'll miss at least a month of school, the time needed to get the disease under control. The main problem right now is one of infection. If you stay free of infection you will be out of the hospital in about five days, if an infection occurs you'll be hospitalized for at least two weeks.

This style of homogenized information giving is likely to be highly ineffective for younger children, and only slightly less so for older children, adolescents and adults. Even where an opportunity exists for questions to follow the monologue, most of the information will have been missed. If the patient recalls anything it is likely to be leukemia and hospital for two weeks. This information should be more structured, using explicit categorisation, and in smaller units, allowing for patient's responses before moving on to the next unit (see Chapter 9).

Sometimes, the health worker may disclose bad news to children about their parent or sibling. For example there may be occasion to mention illness in the mother. Children show a number of coping behaviours when faced with this situation (Issel, Ersek and Lewis, 1990) but most seem to receive help from their families.

Disclosing catastrophic bad news

Catastrophic bad news disclosure is infrequently required but is of such magnitude, either personally or otherwise, that it is likely to have a profound effect on the patient, relatives, or community. These situations are usually unexpected and extensive such as natural or man-made disasters, for example. In such events, whole families can be lost, leaving perhaps one injured survivor. Major traffic accidents remain disturbingly common and informing survivors of the death of their family can be a harrowing experience for anyone. Health workers, police and other emergency workers may have the job of breaking such news. Hopefully, most of us will not have to confront this situation. If you do find yourself in the position of having to disclose this information it will be a difficult task.

A patient who has been injured in an accident, who may have lost consciousness and who is unaware that his or her immediate family have been killed, for example, may ask urgent questions about their whereabouts. This can be particularly difficult if the survivor is a child.

Under these circumstances, next of kin should be identified at the earliest opportunity following admission once the circumstances become known. The police should take care of this, but check this is done. The next of kin may live many miles away or be unidentifiable and the child may need answers.

Loss of parents is particularly difficult for a child to cope with because of the latter's dependency on the adults. It will be painful and the child may feel a profound sense of abandonment and loss, and an overpowering sense of despair, helplessness and threat.

The developmental age of the child will influence the level of information that can be given. A pre-school child in this situation will need close support and counselling for many months. Older children and adolescents will also need this, but are more able to intellectually deal with the event. Younger children may need repeated explanations of why the event occurred. Older children may not need this so much.

Pt: Why haven't my mum and dad come to see me?
HW: They would if they could, I'm sure, but they aren't able to, I'm afraid Louise.
Pt: Why not? What's wrong?

(Health worker takes patient's hand.)

HW: Your mum and dad were hurt very badly in the accident.
Pt: How bad? Are they in hospital too? Are they alright?
HW: Your mum and dad didn't wake up after the accident.
Pt: They're dead?

HW: (Nods)
Pt: Peter . . . ?
HW: Your brother too. I'm so sorry . . .
Pt: Oh no . . . all of them? No! (Patient cries.)

(Health worker puts arms around patient and holds her. Health worker doesn't try to reassure or explain; holding is the only effective act at this stage.)

The sudden, total disclosure is an emotional avalanche. However, a gradual approach may be more difficult to control, and a semi-sudden, semi-gradual partial cum total disclosure may be the result.

This scene may be different if the child denies the news. The child may become angry and even try to leave the hospital. Under these circumstances, the enormity of the event is too much for the child to deal with.

A controlled release of information may be best until the level of coping is accurately assessed. The nature of the event is bound to make coping extremely difficult for the child. Long-term counselling support will almost certainly be needed.

The spouse of a parent who has died suddenly, such as in a traffic accident, may feel unable to cope with personal grief and the demands of the grieving child. Close counselling support will be mandatory for this family.

Disclosure in obstetric situations

There are several special situations in obstetrics, paediatrics and genetics where the importance of disclosure may be overlooked or played down. However, these areas are important and should be handled as the more obvious situations, with telling a diagnosis, prognosis or other unexpected result.

Informing a couple about inter-uterine or perinatal death

The death of a child before birth is a source of distress and guilt to the parents, especially the mother. The circumstances surrounding the pregnancy may be important. A couple trying to have a baby for many years will likely feel profound disappointment; a sense of failure may occur even for a woman carrying an unwanted child. An inter-uterine death occurring early during the first trimester of pregnancy will probably cause less distress than one occurring during the third trimester (Theut, Zaslow, Rabinovich, Bartko and Morihisa, 1990) though this should not be assumed. Death occurring during birth or in the few days following birth (perinatal death) can be equally or more traumatic for the parents (Menke and McClead, 1990).

The mother is vulnerable to powerful feelings of failure and guilt about the death. The death implicitly accuses her of an inability to provide a nurturing womb for her child to grow. It challenges a fundamental aspect of her womanhood. It threatens to expose her as a failure both biologically and socially to fulfill what many women view as a key role within their lives (Weiss, Frischer and Richman, 1989; Layne, 1990). Some spouses feel as profound a sense of loss as the mother (Theut et al, 1990).

The process of disclosure about inter-uterine or perinatal death can be helped by an understanding of the circumstances surrounding the pregnancy. Is it the first pregnancy of a young couple, or a late attempt to have a child by a couple who have had fertility difficulties? What were the circumstances of the death? It has been estimated that between 20% to 30% of all pregnancies end with inter-uterine or perinatal death (Layne, 1990). Causes may result from illness or non-viability of the child, miscarriage, birth trauma, termination due to genetic disease, prematurity and other reasons.

Until recently, it was rarely possible for parents of a mature, stillborn or days-old baby who had died to even see the child, let alone hold and be with the baby. The last 15 years has seen a tendency to acknowledge and attempt to prevent the significant psychological distress that occurs when parents are separated from the infant, and the death is 'swept under the carpet' (Zeaneh, 1989).

Such parents may continue to experience difficulties in having their loss recognized as a legitimate loss of a child, and themselves as bereaved parents. Instead, terms like embryo, fetus and neonate used by health workers depersonalize (and thereby de-emotionalize) the event. A second problem faced by parents and family, is one of confusion and uncertainty (Layne, 1990): Why has the event happened? Explanations may not be forthcoming.

A failure of health workers to deal effectively with the death can impair parental and family adjustment. This can result in severe complications: depression, psychosis for mothers, mainly following the next live birth; family disagreement; disturbances, running away, drug use, or suicide among already born or future children, especially for a subsequent 'replacement' child (Rousseau, 1988). More commonly, less extreme but persistent grieving occurs (Murray and Callan, 1988).

Parents of multiple birth, one or more of whom die may be vulnerable to a mix of confusing feelings; joy for the survivors, grief for the dead (Swanson-Kauffman, 1988). By allowing parents to interact with the dead child(ren), they can more readily adjust to the care of the surviving siblings.

To facilitate adaptation to the loss, it is important to allow the parents to hold and touch the child. Support from staff is also recognized as vital to good care (Rousseau, 1988; Murray and Callan, 1988). Being with the baby is important for the formation of a few memories the parents could keep, and facilitates greater satisfaction with care and higher parental self-esteem (Murray and Callan, 1988). Support from staff also increases satisfaction with care, parental self-esteem and adjustment (Murray and Callan, 1988).

It seems to be important to disclose the situation as soon as possible in the case of inter-uterine death, and to see the couple jointly where possible. This minimizes uncertainty and prepares the couple for the process of expelling the dead child. For the same reasons, it seems advisable that in the case of unexpected stillbirth, disclosure should take place with the minimum of delay. This is likely to be in the delivery room.

Disclosure should be truthful and full. The parents should be encouraged to be with the dead child if stillborn or days-old. For an earlier term baby, this should also be done, if the parents want it. However, do not force the parents if they resist this suggestion. The health worker should be prepared to listen and answer any questions. Except for acts to maintain the mother's physical well-being, priority should be given to help the parents cope with their disappointment and shock. Encouraging the expression of emotion is usually helpful. That disclosure should be done with sensitivity goes without saying. Avoid referring to the baby as 'it'; where the gender is know, use he or she as appropriate and the name if one is decided on.

Example:

HW: Mrs Jones, Mr Jones, I'm terribly sorry to have to tell you, but as you suspected, your baby is not moving.

Mo: I knew it. There's something gone wrong, isn't there?

HW: We are not able to find a heartbeat.

Mo: No heartbeat?

HW: We don't think so, no. It seems that her heart has stopped.

Fa: Is it, . . . it's dead?

HW: Yes, I'm afraid so. I'm very sorry. I know this must be a terrible shock to you, but there is nothing that can be done in these circumstances.

Mo: But what . . . what happened? It was alright. My doctor said everything was alright. What happened?

HW: We don't know. Sometimes this happens for reasons that we don't fully understand. It happens quite suddenly, like a heart attack.

Fa: Oh, Sue . . . .(Puts arms around the mother; hold each other).

(Health worker remains silent, but 'with' the couple.)

Fa: What's going to happen..?
HW: We think the baby should be born within the next 24 hours. We will give some drugs to help labour begin.
Mo: Labour, with nothing at the end.
HW: I expect it seems awful. We'll do what we can to make it quick.
Mo: Yes, I don't want it, I don't even know what it is, I don't want her dead, staying inside me.
HW: Of course not. I'll leave you to be together for a while. Once again, I'm sorry this has happened to you. If there's anything I or the other staff can do, just ask.

Following the initial disclosure, parents may later seek information on when or if it is safe to embark on another pregnancy at some time. Parents seem to resent being given advice on this and should be given information, not instruction, being allowed to decide for themselves (Davis, Stewart and Harmon, 1989).

As a final point, many hospitals now put families bereaved by perinatal death in contact with support groups or run such groups themselves.

Genetic counselling and related situations

A second set of circumstances which may be closely related to the aetiology of perinatal death is the problem of genetic disorders. A neonate with an identified genetic syndrome may be stillborn or live only a few days in severe cases. Thus, coping with a neonatal death may be exacerbated if there is a need to counsel the parents about future children.

Where the child survives, or where there is the identification of genetic disorder in older family members, the need to disclose to the family important relevant information arises. The matter may be more complex than simply disclosing information. In order to identify or confirm a disorder, or identify its inheritance pattern, detailed information may be required of the family. This may involve all surviving relatives, with requests for access to photographs and other family information, including physical or other examinations (Onadim, Hykin, Hungerford and Cowell, 1991). In other words, the enquiries can be particularly penetrating.

This type of enquiry should be left until the parents have had a reasonable length of time to come to terms with their loss.

Disclosing the suspicion of a serious genetic disorder can be very disruptive to a family. Where the condition is sex-linked, future pregnancies can be screened to identify the sex of the baby and then a decision can be made whether to proceed with the pregnancy or not. Where there is no sex-linkage, then children who themselves are not sufferers of the disease may be carriers. This may bring its own set of problems that these children will need to be informed and to make adaptations later.

For some disorders, expression of the condition does not occur until later life, e.g. Huntington's chorea; familial colorectal cancers, which comprise about 40% of all colorectal cancers (Bodmer et al, 1989). Children may be susceptible to the disease in later life. Young adults planning a family may need to take their own genetic status into account.

In other disorders, two copies of the gene (homozygous) must be present for the disease to appear. If only one partner carries the affected gene, all children will be unaffected (though some may also be carriers). More difficult to predict and counsel against are what are known as heterogeneous disorders (where hereditary diseases is due to mutation at different gene sites: human chromosomes have several copies of any given gene). Under these circumstances, it can be very difficult for the genetic counsellor to advise families of individual probability of risk (Narod, 1991).

A further problem is the difficulty in arriving at a diagnosis. Early in life, it may be difficult to diagnose some conditions with the result that health worker uncertainty will be high. Some diagnoses will be made post-natally, but which need to be corrected as the child grows. Parents may be unwilling to accept that the genetic explanation is correct and the 'environmental' (and often socially less stigmatizing) cause is not valid (Tse, Temple and Baraitser 1990; Hiew and Lim, 1991).

Thus, the information involved in disclosing bad news can often be technical and complex, with varying levels of uncertainty.

Cultural explanations may take prominence over genetic explanations for disease. This can be particularly problematic in traditional and closely knit communities. Many minority communities have high levels of genetic disorders due to inter-marriage to strengthen family ties (consanguineous marriages). The frequency of mutant genes, and thus genetic disorders can be high compared to more heterogeneous communities (Wright, 1990; Jaruzelska et al, 1991; Janson, Jayakoddy, Abulaban and Gustavson, 1991). This has several consequences for disclosing bad news to members of minority groups who have particularly traditional attitudes. First, the explanation may be rejected in favour of a more traditional view (Wright, 1990). This can make it problematic for the counsellor trying to advise families. This is an important example of why the patient's interpretation of events and world view should be consulted first (see Chapters 2 and 3). A second consequence may be that if the genetic explanation is accepted, certain members of a family may become victimized as a result. These are likely to be females who have come into the family by marriage, and who may be seen as tainted or inadequate (Carmi, 1991). These women also tend to be blamed if there is infertility, despite the fact that the husband is as likely to be infertile as the woman.

These points should be borne in mind in preparing for disclosure of this kind of information and care needs to be taken in avoiding further family disruption.

Disclosure should, as always, be open and straightforward. In genetic counselling, written information can be particularly useful to explain simple varieties of inheritance. Several contacts may need to be made with different members of the family. Where cooperation is required, it is important not to underestimate the importance of support and empathic behaviour towards the family.

An important point has been made that 'the offer of prenatal diagnosis implies a recommendation to accept that offer, which in turn implies a tacit recommendation to terminate a pregnancy if it is found to show any abnormality. I believe that this sequence is present irrespective of the counsellor's wishes, thoughts or feelings, because it arises from the social context rather than from the personalities involved' (Clarke, 1991). This is clearly very important and as Clarke points out, great care needs to be taken to avoid compounding this implicit pressure to terminate 'abnormal' pregnancy with a non-supportive attitude from the health worker.

Summary

- The patient has the right to know or to not know bad news, and the health worker has the primary responsibility as the informer to see this need is met.
- Assess patient readiness for information by spending some time in discussion beforehand.
- Disclose bad news in a private and supportive environment, making preparation for the need to disclose before the patient begins to request information: information management.
- Withholding information is not protecting the patient, and usually leads to difficult situations between the staff and patient.
- The patient has a right to honest and full information in order to effectively plan for the future. Failure to provide this if the patient requests it may be considered unethical.
- Be aware of the difficulties patients may have in getting the opportunity to ask questions: provide opportunities in which patients can, if they wish, feel free to ask difficult questions.

- Using the full disclosure and mop-up approach requires preparation of information and time to deal with the reactions to the news.
- Using step-wise approach allows greater control over the information being disclosed, but may be more difficult in other ways.
- Children need to know what is happening to them just as adults do, perhaps more so. Information must be given in such a way as to be meaningful to the child.
- In neonatal death, encourage parents to spend time with the dead infant.

Exercises

1. *Situation:* The mother (or father) of a child (decide now on appropriate age for the participant) has been asked to meet the health worker and discuss the child patient's condition. The child has been hospitalised for two days following signs of sudden behaviour disturbance and partial blindness of the right side.

   You are the health worker. The mother does not know yet that the child has an confirmed brain tumour, called an astrocytoma. This type of tumour is malignant and will kill the child unless surgery and chemotherapy are performed without delay. The tumour is located in the left hemisphere of the brain (the side associated with language). Surgery will involve removal of a large part of the left hemisphere of the brain. The drug treatment afterwards could also cause brain damage, but is necessary to kill any remaining cancer cells.

   Success with the operation is high, around 90%. However, there is a strong chance that the child will be brain damaged. His language ability is almost certain to be seriously affected. If the child is young, aged less than five, chances for recovery of some language function are moderate; if older than five, they are poor.

   You are the parent. This boy/girl (think of a name and use it) is the eldest of two children. He or she was a bright and outgoing child until about two weeks ago when a teacher reported that the child's school work deteriorated badly. You noticed the child began to get clumsy and aggressive. You consulted your GP who arranged for the child to come into hospital for 'tests'.

Your spouse works in a clerical job, and you have a part time job for a bit of extra money. Your relationship with your spouse is fair, but not as good as you would like.

You are a believer in medical care, but not at any cost to the patient. Otherwise, be yourself.

Task: To disclose the diagnosis and discuss the implications with the parent.
Time available: 15 minutes.

2. *Situation:*   A hospital emergency area has recently admitted a young female aged 25 years following an hit-and-run road accident. The next of kin, a sister/brother, has been contacted and has just arrived at the hospital. It is 9.30 p.m.

You are health worker.   The patient was dead on arrival. The cause is multiple trauma due to a hit-and-run road accident. The driver has not yet been found. Police have contacted the home address. They have brought the next-of-kin who is a younger/older brother/sister. The parents are away on vacation and the two siblings have no other relatives in town.

You are the relative.   You are the younger (older) daughter (son) in a four member family, with an older (younger) sister aged 25, and your mother and father. Your parents have gone away for a week's holiday leaving you and your sister on your own for the first time. Your sister went out at about 8.00 p.m. to meet a friend. Ten minutes ago, the police knocked at your door. All they would tell you is that your sister had 'been in an accident' and that they would take you to the hospital. You are now waiting to see the health worker to be told what has happened. You are close to your sister and understandably very worried. Otherwise, be yourself.

Task: Health worker to explain the circumstances of the accident and consequences to the relative.
Time available: 10 minutes.

3. *Situation:*   Patient is in hospital for exploration of weight loss.

You are the health worker.   You are a senior member of staff on a medical/surgical ward in a busy general hospital. The patient in question is the spouse of your partner in this exercise. They have a ten-week history of weight loss. A body scan earlier today identified a 3 cm tumour of the left lung, with a large (8 cm) tumour of the liver. A provisional diagnosis of hepatocellular carcinoma (cancer of the liver) with secondaries in the left lung has been made.

The ward is very busy today and there are two members of your team off sick. The spouse of the patient has asked to talk to you. You think it is important to tell the patient of the diagnosis, given the patient's relatively young age. There is the possibility of some radical treatment (surgery and chemotherapy). Otherwise, be yourself. The patient has asked indirectly one of the junior nurses.

You are the relative.   Your spouse was admitted to hospital for two days of tests because he or she had been losing weight for about three months. Your spouse does not cope very well in crises. No one has told you anything and you have asked to talk with the health worker. You are concerned that it is something serious, like cancer. If it is a serious condition, you do not want your spouse to be told because you don't think he or she could cope with the news.

Task: To decide what to tell the patient.
Time available: To be negotiated, but no more than 15 minutes.

Discussion

1. What factors should a health worker take into consideration when deciding what to tell children under five about a chronic non-fatal illness?

2. If the parents of a six-year-old child refuse to tell the child of a fatal diagnosis, should the health worker give this information despite the parents' wishes? If so, why? If not, why not?

3. How would you handle the refusal of a patient to accept a bad news diagnosis involving a fatal illness?

4. Can you think of other ways to disclose bad news, than those two given in this chapter? If you use other ways to disclose, why do you prefer those ways? Discuss with your group the advantages and disadvantages of different disclosure strategies.

12

Pain and Communications With the Dying

Educational Objectives

By the end of this chapter, you should be able to

- list the important features of the human loss reaction
- recognize ambivalent feelings in the dying person
- describe causes of premature abandonment of dying patients
- describe the contribution of uncertainty to distress and anxiety and thereby to adjustment in the dying patient
- discuss the perceptual nature of pain and limitations of traditional methods of pain control for the dying and give an account of the intensification of pain due to depression and anxiety
- recognize the need for effective and appropriate pain control during terminal illness and describe the role of communication in pain control
- give examples of staff distancing tactics in the care of the dying and recognize the need to spend time with the dying
- describe and identify different levels of awareness of dying
- describe the benefits to patients relatives/friends of open communications and interactions with the dying
- give an account of the principal needs of dying children and adolescents
- describe how to communicate effectively with dying children and their family
- recognize the importance of whole-family care in the care of dying children
- identify major components of communications used with dying children
- demonstrate appropriate techniques for communicating with the dying and the bereaved

▓ Introduction

> Our last garment is made without pockets.
>
> Italian proverb

So far, we have considered problems occurring in various health care situations. This chapter deals with communications during illness about dying, communications during the patient's decline, and communications with the bereaved after death has occurred.

This chapter contains some material that may initially appear unrelated to clinical communications skills. However, it is a key tenet of this book that health care approaches fundamentally communicate how we value and care for others. In other words, communication is *implied* whether intended or not, in the global range of behaviour we call health care. For this reason, two major topics of current importance in health care today are discussed in the context of this chapter. These are cancer and pain: cancer because it remains for many the most feared form of death, and pain because it is such an important symptom generally and specifically in cancer. Since dying is a major issue for most people, these two areas are discussed as topics for care in a wider context of care for the dying. The techniques section of this chapter still focuses on aspects of communication techniques for use with dying patients. Dying is the area that staff seem to report most difficulty in dealing with, and pain control is among the most important contribution health care has to make in care of the dying. For these reasons, this chapter may be perceived more as a focus on management of pain and dying, than on a more narrow definition of communication skills technique. But it should be seen as both.

The meaning of death from cancer

The choice of placing this section in the present chapter was a hard one because it contradicts the point that many people with cancer recover completely. Only 38% of patients with cancers survive more than five years, thus there is more dread attached to cancers than almost any other illness, perhaps with the current exception of AIDS. Circulatory diseases have twice the mortality rate of cancers, and are the leading causes of death in most industrialized countries (Taylor and Crisler, 1988). Despite this, it is cancer that is feared. 'Cardiac disease implies a weakness, trouble, fatigue that is mechanical: there is no disgrace . . .' (Sontag, 1978), yet cancer implies corruption, decay and evil. It is considered insidious and analogous to death, both by the public and by many health workers.

These meanings result in cancers being viewed as frightening and unique. The major sources of distress for cancer patients are the uncertainty of their medical status, fear of deterioration, the threat of aggressive anti-cancer treatment, and fear of intense pain and an inevitable death (Fishman and Loscalzo, 1987). Turk and Fernandez (1990) argue that it is these assumptions about the meaning of cancer that underlie many of the difficulties in controlling pain in patients with cancer. One can go further, arguing that these beliefs are subtly confirmed by health workers in their different treatment of patients with cancer compared to other patients. As a result, the cancer patient is ascribed a unique status in the nursing and medical literature. This is true, even to the point that patients who are dying from cancer have their own special place to die. It is cancer that is seen most frequently in hospice care. Almost everyone else dies in hospital or at home (Cartwright, Hockey and Anderson, 1978).

The majority of research into dying has been in patients dying from cancer. Patients with cardiac or cerebrovascular disease tend to die in the ICU or on acute medical wards, along with common causes of death associated with other major organ failures. What is it that makes cancers special, if not the metaphor of cancer as evil decay? For the first time since the decline of tuberculosis as a major cause of death in industrialized countries, cancer has a rival, AIDS, which in just over a decade has acquired a greater cultural stigma.

For the remainder of this chapter, care of the dying patient is explored from a communications perspective. It is mostly assumed that the patient in question will be dying from this group of diseases we call cancers. However, the reader is urged to bear in mind that many of the problems and communications difficulties associated with care of the dying are, in most cases, compounded when cancer is the underlying disease. In some cases, the diagnosis of cancer (or AIDS) is the single most important reason for the problems. The previous few paragraphs have outlined the principal reasons for this point of view.

Problems experienced by the dying

> Hardest of deaths to a mortal is the death he sees ahead.
>
> Bacchylides (5th century BC)

There are two certainties in life: death and taxes. Few people face impending death without some sense of the meaning of life. For many, dying starkly defines life and an understanding of death is inherent in living. Death is something we try hard to avoid. Fear of dying motivates sometimes extreme acts, perhaps paradoxically even suicide (Gunnell and

Frankel, 1994). Whether the response to the knowledge of impending death is anxiety, anger, remorse or sadness, few will not grasp hungrily at the opportunity to extend their life. But not at any price. There are times when it is preferable to die than continue to live and requests are increasingly made for assistance to die (Baile et al, 1993). Even then, many cling on. Given the choice of a meaningful life supported by friends and loved ones, few choose death.

Health workers' anxiety about dying can make them feel very uncomfortable in the presence of the dying person, or in discussing the prognosis or death (Martin, 1982). This influences the care dying people receive (Schultz and Aderman, 1979). The consequence is that death anxiety in health workers makes it very difficult for them to function effectively with the dying.

What is it about dying that is so difficult to deal with? There are several components which can be identified, including loss, isolation, fear of pain, fear of the consequences for the self, family and friends.

Loss

> In the depths of anxiety at having to die
> is the anxiety of being eternally forgotten.
>
> Paul Tillich (1963)

The difficulties surrounding dying involve fear of the unknown and loss of consciousness, experience, loved ones, pleasure, the future, and the self.

According to Erikson (1963), adapting to loss is one of the developmental tasks of older adulthood. This involves 'letting go' of the lost object. Giving up feelings invested in the lost object is the purpose of grieving. The greatest loss of all for many is the loss brought on by our own deaths. Not all deaths occur in old age. Death occurring in childhood and young adulthood is seen as a tragedy in some societies, though is expected in many more. For a young person anticipating the (illusionary) advantages of adulthood, only to be deprived while others go on to achieve them, can lead to greater difficulty in adaptation for the dying person and family. There are differences between letting go of the past and letting go of the future.

Adaptation is making sense of what is happening within the context of a person's life experience and world view. Hence, adaptation to the loss of dying impels the person to make sense of an illness or event causing death. The more meaning a person can perceive in an event, then the more understandable it becomes. People who cannot understand or explain to themselves their ending lives may experience greater difficulty in resolving their feelings over dying.

Loss is frequently associated with depression, probably due to an inability to return that which is lost (Bowlby, 1972). It follows that adaptation to loss may also help to resolve depressive responses seen earlier in the adaptation process, and conversely, failure to adapt may bring increasing distraught and helpless experiences.

Separation from loved ones occurs temporarily during hospitalization and permanently at death. This occurs at a time when the desire for closeness, love and protection may be evoked at high levels by the patient's circumstances. The dying person is different from the healthy. The dying person is slipping away and nothing can alter this fact. There is helplessness and anticipatory grief in relatives who may begin the process of letting go of the dying patient.

Thus, the dying person may have an ambivalent need for closeness and support while simultaneously feeling increasingly isolated from others. Loss of previous roles and the perception of the self as a liability may cause misery to the dying person. The patient may not want to feel responsible for the grief seen in others (Hinton, 1967).

This ambivalence of feeling is marked in the period of adaptation to dying. There may be a strong need to talk about the event and the experience, but others may find this off-putting, perceiving it as morbid or depressing, and urge the person to talk about 'brighter things', and to 'try and cheer up'. This may be punctuated with periods of withdrawal where despite efforts by others, the dying person resists attempts to be drawn in to the social milieu (Hinton, 1967). Similarly, relatives may withdraw from the dying person too (Kalish, 1966). This mutual moving apart and coming together may not be synchronous, and at times one or the other may feel abandoned or crowded.

The health workers involved in caring for seriously ill and dying patients needs to be aware of these feelings in planning communications care. Information becomes very important, but a shift in priorities is also needed — towards spending time with the person. Health workers need to abandon the perception that spending time with patients is not 'real' work.

Most people have some anxieties about dying and death, though the frequency of anxiety about dying far outweighs that about death (Hinton, 1967; Lamerton, 1973). Many people are frightened of the process of dying. The main components of this are fear of pain and suffering (Fry, 1990). Levels of anxiety about dying vary but they are present in most of us to some extent. Most are likely to stem from uncertainty.

Many conflicts face the dying person which are part of the adaptation to dying. How does this affect health communications?

One mistaken belief is that one 'doesn't talk about it' for fear of upsetting the person. If dying patients want to talk about their circumstances, then the health professional should *not* change the subject. Often, only listening is needed. Sometimes there will be discussion. Such discussion may be a necessary part of the patients' adjustment to their 'different' condition. Similarly, the opportunity and motivation to socialize should be maintained wherever possible. This should be balanced with a person's desire for periodic withdrawal. Many patients will talk very readily about their thoughts and feelings, if given the opportunity (Hinton, 1967).

Key Points

Adapting to dying involves giving up attachments.

Depression or mood disturbance can occur in reaction to loss. Adaptation to dying should lead to resolution of depression.

Dying patients may have ambivalent feelings about social contact. They may simultaneously feel a need to be closer to others, while at the same time having feelings they want to be alone.

Maintaining hope

The maintenance of hope is important and should be pursued where realistic. There is always room for some hope about something, even in late stage terminal illness. Most terminally ill patients are able to retain high levels of hope, with the exception of patients with AIDS (Herth, 1990). This may have much to do with the contemporary image of AIDS as a plague for which there is no cure (Black, 1986; Dozor and Meece, 1990). There remains a moralistic, and in some cases biblical sense of judgement associated with AIDS, despite public education to the contrary (Black, 1986).

Premature abandonment

> It has often been said that it is not death,
> but dying, which is terrible.
>
> Henry Fielding (1751)

The previous section on adaptation to loss presupposed that patients knew their diagnosis, and in the early stages of adaptation would attempt to make sense of it by fitting it into their own frame of reference. However, it is by no means the case that patients are given honest and open diagnoses, or, particularly, prognoses in diseases when the prognoses are poor (Fielding, Ko and Wong, 1995). The undesirable consequences of withholding information on diagnosis and prognosis in circumstances where the patient desires information need consideration.

The diagnosis and prognosis are usually known by the health worker before being made known to the patient. Often, the relatives are first to be told the diagnosis and, perhaps, prognosis (Holdaway, 1985, Fielding et al, 1994), probably more so if the patient is a child. Some health professionals feel that their task of disclosure is done when they have told the relatives (Fielding et al, 1994). It may go no further than that, or there may be later disclosure to the patient. Many relatives try to protect the patient from being upset and ask the doctor 'not to tell' the patient (Gilhooly et al, 1988). Staff may agree to this (Youll, 1989), but not always (Fielding et al, 1994).

Social death

The consequences of witholding desired information can be tragic. In a 'worst case' situation, the following may happen: The relative makes a request to withhold the nature of the illness from the patient. The doctor agrees. The doctor or senior nurse instructs the other staff not to inform the patient of the diagnosis.

Later, when the patient asks a question of a nurse about the condition, the trap created is sprung: if the nurse answers honestly, she disobeys the orders; if she doesn't she must lie or evade the patient's request. Moreover, because responding with evasion or lies is understandably uncomfortable for the nursing staff, the best strategy is to avoid situations where the patient will ask such questions. To do this, staff either avoid interaction with the patient wherever possible, or, when with the patient avoid all talk of diagnosis, change the subject, or ignore all together any related topics (Martin, 1982). As junior nurses carry out the majority of nursing care, spending most time with patients, they are most likely to be asked about diagnosis and prognosis by the patient. As they are the least experienced at evading patient requests, this can be very stressful and staff avoid this by avoiding the patient.

So the patient is isolated as staff try to avoid the patient. Relatives and friends reassure, ignore, or change the subject, as do staff, whenever the issue of diagnosis or prognosis is raised by the patient. The patient has become the victim of a conspiracy of silence, the goal of which is to withhold from the patient the true nature of the illness.

There are many ways this may come about, but the end result is the same for the patient — social death, isolation at the time when the patient needs increased support from family, friends and staff. These good intentions of well-meaning relatives and staff only add to the patient's uncertainty.

High levels of uncertainty make predicting demands very difficult. This reduces the patient's sense of perceived control over threat, increasing coping demand. The patient is then more likely to experience stress and anxiety. Simultaneously, the patient is isolated and more prone to bodily preoccupation due to lack of distraction and shrinkage of the perceptual field. This affects the appraisal of bodily sensations and other symptoms, while anxiety lowers the patient's threshold for labeling sensory events as pain rather than emotional distress (Pennebaker, 1982).

Isolation also makes communication about physical discomfort difficult. There are persistent shortcomings in pain assessment by staff (Cartwright, 1985; Carr, 1990; Fielding, 1994). Increased isolation of the patient complicates accurate pain assessment. Inadequate pain assessment makes inappropriate analgesia more likely.

Staff expect patients with cancer to have 'cancer pain', and so they too label distress as pain (it is more understandable and there are 'treatments') (Turk and Fernandez, 1990). Additionally, physical discomfort, especially that we call pain, contributes to depression (Hinton, 1967). Depression leads to greater self-absorption, contributing still further to the level of suffering.

Increased anxiety and depression contribute to the intensification of pain. More powerful drug regimens attempt to control this pain, resulting in clouding of consciousness and loss of competence, more emotional distress, more drugs, and so on, in a vicious cycle. If drugs are not given, the patient suffers with high levels of pain. The patient often dies alone, wretched and lacking the opportunity to put life in order and depart with dignity. Effective palliative care prevents this (Davis and Hardy, 1994).

Preventing social death

The prevention of social death should be a priority in care of the dying. It is in most cases simple to achieve.

1. Relatives may ask that diagnostic or prognostic information be withheld from the patient.
2. When this happens the health worker should gently acknowledge the understandability of the relative's desire to avoid the patient's suffering.
3. The health worker might discuss with the relatives their reasons for wanting to withhold the information. (Use the reflective techniques discussed in previous chapters.)

Relatives may not want the patient's remaining time to be 'spoilt' by the knowledge of impending death. They should be informed that patients usually end up suffering more if they are not told. They may also believe the patient will 'not be able to cope' with such bad news, or that the patient would 'give up'. In both cases it can be pointed out to the relatives that very few patients are unable to cope if given love and support from their families and staff. There does seem to be a point at which patients accept the inevitable, but others do not (Hinton, 1967). In contrast, some patients become very strongly determined to fight the disease and make substantial changes to their lives to try and achieve this. There is some evidence this may help to prolong survival (Greer, Morris and Pettingale, 1979), but this evidence remains equivocal (Morris, Greer, Watson and Pettingale, 1981).

4. The relatives should then be told, gently but firmly, that the first responsibility of the health worker is to the patient.
5. This being the case, the health worker is obliged to take cue from the patient.

Discussion with the relatives can provide pointers to expectations of patients for information. However, the final decision should always be based on information from the patient.

Schain (1990) states, 'Although public testimony often conveys the conviction that physician communications are limited or altered in an attempt to protect patients from emotional upset and that withholding information is in their best interest, a literature review demonstrated that this was not so. Interestingly, today, a contrary trend may be emerging, where some physicians are so forthright and blunt in their disclosure that the impact of a guarded prognosis is felt as an assault and carries with it a connotation of certainty for disaster.' This, it goes without saying, must be avoided too.

Thus, there is no excuse to withhold information on these grounds. Indeed, involvement of relatives in the care of patients seems to be beneficial in helping both to adapt to the situation. Generally, interaction is more productive and adaptive than isolation or exclusion of relatives.

It is important that an evaluation of the patient's information needs is made early on in the contact with the patient. This cannot be over emphasized as one of the most important aspects of effective communications care of those thought or known to be terminally ill.

> ## Key Points
>
> Withholding information from dying patients who want informa-
> tion on their condition often leads to uncertainty and social
> isolation. This is sometimes called 'social death'.
>
> Distress generated by uncertainty in the patient can increase pain
> experience and make pain control much more difficult. As a result
> the patient may be sedated and unable to function effectively.
>
> Unnecessary distress leads to unnecessary medication, which may
> strip the patient of independence and dignity.

Pain

This topic has great importance in health care. Pain is among the most
common symptoms people report and is a major reason for seeking health
care. Pain is defined by the International Association for the Study of Pain
(IASP) as 'an unpleasant sensory and emotional experience associated
with actual or potential tissue damage, or described in terms of such
damage.' Importantly, the IASP definition goes on '. . . Activity induced in
the nociceptor and nociceptive pathways by a noxious stimulus *is not
pain*, which is always a psychological state, even though we may well
appreciate that pain most often has a proximate physical cause' (Mersky,
1986) (author's emphasis).

Pain is one of the most feared aspects of illness. Pain also makes other
things difficult to bear. In acute illness or injury, pain signals tissue damage. In more chronic conditions, pain becomes ambiguous. It does not
signal new tissue damage yet it persists. Coupled with some incurable
diseases, like certain forms of cancer, it '. . . is all-embracing, unremitting
and destructive' (Hanratty, 1983). This is the classical view of pain, and
the prevailing stereotype of cancer pain. But just how accurate is such a
definition?

Moderate to severe pain was assessed as present in 40% to 45% of
patients initially following a diagnosis of cancer, in 35% to 40% of
patients at intermediate stages of the disease (perhaps representing a decrease in numbers experiencing pain as adaptation to the implication of
the disease occurs), and in 60% to 85% of those with advanced cancer
(Bonica,1984).

Chronic and unremitting pain can be avoided in almost all cases
according to Hanratty (1983). If so, it is a major indictment of the care

given to dying people that pain continues to be the most frequent complaint experienced by dying patients (Cartwright, Hockey and Anderson, 1973; Hanratty, 1983; Cleeland, 1987). Pain is the major cause of depression in dying patients, and continues to be a key cause of anxiety about dying (Hinton, 1967; Cartwright, Hockey and Anderson, 1973; Fry, 1990). And therein lies the problem.

Traditional approaches to pain control have limitations. These include:

- poor assessment of pain level in patients (Cartwright, 1985; Carr, 1990; Fielding, 1994)
- low correlation between pain levels and analgesia dosage (Cartwright, 1985)
- limited efficacy of drugs, restrictions on permitted dosages or on pathways of administration (Cleeland, 1987)
- side-effects of narcotic analgesics needed for pain control including constipation, nausea, vomiting and even respiratory distress
- undue fear remains among physicians about drug dependence and addiction (Foley, 1985)
- rapid tolerance to narcotic and other analgesics means that these drugs may need to be 'held in reserve' for later stages of the disease (Murphy, 1973)
- clouding of consciousness soon occurs when narcotic analgesics are given in increasing doses to overcome this rapidly developing tolerance (Siegel, 1975, 1977)
- neuro-surgical techniques do not provide lasting pain relief, with only 30% of patients reporting relief one year after spinal cordotomies (Sundaresan and DiGiancinto, 1988)
- neuro-surgical approaches to pain control can have serious side-effects; bilateral cordotomies can cause bladder dysfunction (30%), disabling disorders of sensation (5%), and death (5%); rhizotomies can result in loss of tactile sense, and chemical hypophysectomies (destruction of pituitary gland) can cause diabetes insipidus and cranial nerve palsies (Sundaresan and DiGiancinto, 1988)
- administration of opiates has on occasion been reported to intensify pain ('paradoxical pain') (Davis and Hardy, 1994)

Turk and Fernadez (1990) challenge three key assumptions about cancer that, they argue, are significant in affecting how cancer is perceived by both patients and health workers. These assumptions are causal in generating the high levels of anxiety and distress that cancer evokes in people's minds. The removal of this anxiety is, in turn, needed to facilitate more adaptive attitudes and behaviours for understanding and coping with pain. Turk and Fernadez's (1990) critique of these assumptions bears close scrutiny.

The first assumption challenged is that cancer is inevitably lethal. This has already been put into perspective with the mortality rates of other diseases. 'Cancer' includes over 100 different diseases, some with very high cure rates, others with poor cure rates. This variability is often obscured for the patient.

The second assumption challenged is that cancer is inevitably painful. For most people, cancer is synonymous with pain and pain is synonymous with infinite suffering. This is one of our most primitive fears (Wellisch, 1981). Anxieties about cancer and dying feature suffering or pain as a primary concern (Levin, Clelland and Dar, 1985; Fry, 1990; Davis and Hardy, 1994). Turk and Fernandez (1990) argued that the assumption of equating cancer with pain is by no means justified. They quote Turnbull's (1979) report that 29% of lung cancer patients experienced little or no pain throughout the course of their disease. Also cited is Ahles, Ruckdeschel and Blanchard's (1984) report that 82% of a sample of lymphoma pa- tients reported no pain, and that of 208 ambulatory cancer patients, only 33.5% had pain due to the disease process, 6.7% had pain from cancer- related surgery, 11% had pain from non- cancerous sources, and 48% did not complain of pain at all.

Third, Turk and Fernandez (1990) challenge the view of pain as uniquely linked to the physical damage of cancer. They argue that, con- trary to the belief that cancer pain is commonly distinguished from other types of non-malignant pain on the basis of its supposed organicity (Levy, 1987/1988), it is intrinsically no different from other types of chronic pain. Any difference between the pain of cancer and other chronic pain is that the cultural meaning of cancer is one which condemns its victims to pain, suffering and almost certain death. It is this unique meaning which is responsible for the high anxiety and depression, which in turn precipi- tates the suffering of cancer.

While there clearly are patients who experience high levels of pain, the extensive literature which fails to show a direct relationship between tissue damage and pain experience in non-malignant disease is seldom considered in the management of cancer. The evidence supporting this contention can be divided into four groups (Turk and Fernandez, 1990):
1. the occurrence of tissue damage not accompanied by pain, such as spinal degeneration in aging
2. the spontaneous occurrence of pain in the absence of identifiable tissue damage, such as causalgia and phantom limb pain (Melzack and Wall, 1982)
3. the distortion of pain by psychological processes, such as situation (Beecher, 1946), reinforcement (Fordyce, 1976), observational learn- ing (Craig, 1986), and other processes
4. the inconsistencies in levels of pain reported by patients before and

after they are diagnosed as having cancer (Black, 1975; Woodforde and Fielding, 1970; Cassell, 1982)

These arguments of Turk and Fernandez are significant enough to warrant repetition here.

Chapter 2 explored the central nature of perception and appraisal processes, with examples related to pain. Turk and Fernandez (1990) identified four main *psychological influences* implicated in the perception and reporting of pain. These are expectancy, distress, symptom meaning, and perceived controllability.

Expectancy

People with cancer, as we have seen, are anticipating an agonizing, evil and lethal experience. By manipulating those expectancies using psychological interventions, a reduction in perceived pain can be achieved. Beecher (1946) demonstrated this with soldiers injured in battle, few of whom required analgesia. He later reported that saline injections, presented as morphine, produced pain relief in about 35% of subjects (Beecher, 1961). Turk and Fernandez (1990) cited an unreferenced study by Yonemoto (1975), who reportedly achieved complete relief of pain for at least four hours in 77% of advanced cancer patients from pharmacological preparations containing no analgesic medication.

Distress

Pain behaviour is both a function of cultural influence (Zboroski, 1969), and of arousal level (Sternbach, 1976). Anxiety increases both the subjective distress and the expressed behaviour associated with pain. The anxiety itself may arise from sources other than the pain, such as relationship problems, fear of dying or frustration over some important goal. A major cause of anxiety is pain and the uncertainty patients may have about whether they can tolerate this. Reassurance of thorough and effective pain control should be explicitly made early on in discussions with the patient. This should be followed through by the health worker.

Anxiety also occupies mental capacity. It can tie up large amounts of the human information processing system, making normal function, such as communication, decision making, learning and memory much less efficient (Williams et al, 1988). Preoccupation with pain may serve a similar purpose with the result that not only is suffering increased, but the vicious cycle generated leaves little room for effective function. Greater dependency and loss of dignity can quickly follow.

Among the seriously ill and dying, depression occurs as a result of deterioration, loss of function or body parts, changes in appearance, and, most significantly, pain (Hinton, 1967; Cartwright, Hockey and Anderson, 1973). Chronic pain is particularly important as a cause of depression. Depression seems to have an even greater interference effect on cognitive function than anxiety (Williams et al, 1988). When cognitive capacity is tied up by anxiety or depression, adaptive coping could take much longer to occur.

Failure to control depression compounds the problems faced by dying patients and severely limits their ability to cope with other aspects of dying. Adaptation becomes difficult under such circumstances.

Meaning of symptoms

How an individual appraises an event determines the meaning it has and that person's subsequent emotional arousal and behaviour. Cancer patients often are isolated which can result in preoccupation with and sensitization to bodily sensations. These sensations serve as a reminder of the disease (and its connotations), and can be interpreted or misinterpreted as pain. The sensations than signify disease progress (Ahles et al, 1983) and cause panic, turning even low intensity discomfort into unbearable pain (Cassell, 1982). (See also Chapters 2 and 3.)

Perceived controllability

Clinical studies on the effects of increasing personal controllability over pain by allowing patients control over analgesia administration have achieved impressive results. Cancer patients receiving bone marrow transplantation who were given control over an infusion pump administering morphine used only 33% of the morphine compared to an equivalent group who were given morphine by a nurse (Hill, Saeger and Chapman, 1986). There is an extensive literature on patient-administered analgesia.

The implications of this material are that in order to effectively care for dying patients, it is not sufficient to simply address biological factors of disease control.

Communicating about dying means considering the psychological processes that are important in human behaviour. Pain behaviour provides a strong communications medium. The crying and moaning of someone in severe pain, the facial expression accompanying injury all in themselves seem to serve no other purpose than social signalling. This indicates the need for help, communicating distress. In other words, much pain behaviour has a social role. And people respond to this behaviour. These responses legitimize and reinforce pain behaviour (Turk and Fernandez, 1990).

Coping with chronic pain may be partly determined by the degree to which the individual accepts that suffering is inevitable (Kotarba, 1983). In the West, the Judeo-Christian belief that suffering is in some way a payment or necessary for the shedding of 'sin' encourages such a view. Learning to live with suffering ('you must learn to live with your pain') can only occur if it can be given meaning within the patient's belief system. Many religions and philosophies provide just such belief systems. These facilitate coping with the stress of life in an uncertain and hazardous world. A viable belief system, such as religion, may make coping with chronic pain more tolerable, or make diseases like cancer more easy to accept, but religion is no substitute for effective pain control.

Key Points

Pain is not simply a product of tissue damage, though sensation may be.

Cancer diagnosis evokes fear of suffering which raises anxiety.

Anxiety intensifies pain experience and is a significant contributor to pain during terminal illness.

Uncontrolled pain is the major cause of depression in dying patients.

Anxiety and depression use up coping capacity that could otherwise be used to help adapt to the diagnosis in a positive manner.

By helping patients re-interpret their experience, considerable reductions in levels of anxiety and in the need for analgesia can be achieved.

Other cognitive-behavioural techniques can add significantly to the management of pain in dying patients.

Pain management

Effective pain control is a crucial aspect in care of the dying. High levels of pain complaint or pain-related behaviour may communicate underlying emotional or mood disturbance such as anxiety or depression. These need to be dealt with directly, and not simply covered up with medication, though such may be very helpful in combination with skilled therapy.

Skilled psychological care is needed to effectively control pain without resorting to high doses of powerful narcotics. This cannot be achieved from a distance and without communication.

What implications does the above discussion have for health professionals' communications with dying patients? Communications with the dying patient should then be as follows:

1. Be open, honest and appropriate to the level desired by the patient; in particular
    *   aim to keep the patient currently informed and consulted over decision making
    *   help maintain where possible a sense of control over, or at very least, involvement in management of the disease
    *   be sensitive and supportive, as appropriate to the patient's needs
2. Consider as major problems for the patient
    *   adaptation to loss
    *   premature abandonment
    *   social isolation or loneliness
    *   pain
    *   anxiety (which is more frequently about fear of pain and dying than about death)
    *   depression, which is more common than anxiety, and usually results from intractable deterioration and poorly controlled pain
3. Wherever possible avoid treating the dying person as a 'patient'. Try where possible to help patients to retain existing roles and responsibilities, and even adoption of new ones is often possible and gives patients a greater sense of control over their lives.
4. Use a cognitive-behavioural perspective in pain management and medication to supplement this.

Special problems faced by health workers caring for dying people

Though it be in the power of the weakest to take away life,
it is not in the strongest to deprive us of death.

Sir Thomas Browne (1642)

Occupational burnout — a state of emotional fatigue — is reportedly a serious problem when there is high patient demand and little positive outcome, such as working in a unit with a high mortality rate (Price and Bergen, 1977). Nursing children or young adults dying from cancer, AIDS, or other progressive diseases can make staff feel they are simply delaying the inevitable. They may be angry with patients who don't fight their diseases; they may be hurt when a special patient dies; they may become emotionally insulated to protect against these demands, but cold as a consequence. What contributes to this burnout?

A major contributor to burnout is the cure-oriented approach of modern health care. The prevailing emphasis on cure in the education of many health professionals, especially physicians and nurses pushes aside education on care, particularly in medical education.

Medical staff are the professional group with the greatest investment in the image of the curer. The emphasis on cure in medical education means that physicians often have difficulty in accepting that dying is as natural as birth. In other words, many members of the medical profession (some of the more hi-tech branches of nursing are beginning to follow suit) periodically lose sight of the fact that death is not a disease and hence has no cure. One result of the focus on cure and control of disease in medical education particularly has been to concentrate the efforts of medicine on curing death. In medical education, hardly any emphasis is placed on care, with the result that the dying patient represents a failure of the curative medical model, and a perception that 'nothing more can be done' once cure is ruled out. The importance given to care of dying in medical education can be gathered from the amount of time given to it in medical curricula. In 1984, an average of only 6.27 hours over five years were spent on formal education about care of the dying in UK medical schools (Field, 1984). Some emphasis on palliative care is now occurring (Davis and Hardy, 1994).

The three C structure of health care

When a patient is defined as 'dying', care tends to shift from medical to nursing staff (Benoliel, 1977). Many medical staff think they have little to offer in care of the dying, and that their time is better spent elsewhere, 'curing'. Yet all medical care can be considered as a three-level hierarchical model; at the top of the pyramid is **cure** of disease, for the few patients who are curable. The bulk of medical education emphasizes cure which constitutes the smallest component of practice. The middle level is **control** of disease. Most medical practice falls into this category. For most diseases other than self-limiting ones, control is all contemporary health care can offer (Thorne, 1993). But the base of the pyramid on which both control and cure rest is **care**. Care is required for all patients, cured, controlled or otherwise. Unfortunately most medical practitioners have never been taught this in medical schools. It is one of the greatest failures of current medical education.

This trend may be changing in the USA. Oncologists at Albany Medical College were found to spend more time with patients with the poorest prognoses. Patient satisfaction with the relationship was found to be high (Blanchard and Ruckdeschel, 1986). However, elsewhere, the most junior medical staff can issue 'do not resuscitate' orders without prior consultation with senior staff, patients or relatives (Candy, 1991), reflecting a withdrawal of more senior staff from the responsibilities of care.

Nursing is only slightly better. Until recently, nursing has focused more on the tasks involved in the physical care of the patient. The patient-oriented care now taught in many nursing education programmes goes a long way to focusing on better psychosocial care. However, the increasing demands to train nurse technologists risk directing nurses' attention away from the person and towards the equipment. Additionally, staff shortages generally mean that tasks continue to get preference over communications, truly a false economy and detrimental to the patient's well-being.

It is worth remembering that there is a belief held by many of the public that hospitals are places where people go when they are sick to be made well again. It seems that many health workers in hospitals also hold similar beliefs (Walsh and Kingston, 1988). This 'hospital philosophy' is contradicted every time a patient dies.

Dying patients frequently communicate failure of curative medicine to nurses as well as doctors (Martin, 1982; Price and Bergen, 1977). It is understandable to want to avoid events which indicate failure. Fortunately, changed practice involving patients more in the decision making about their care is becoming more common, and is crucial at life's end. Recently, attempts have been made to quantify levels of care for dying patients and choices about cardiopulmonary resuscitation. One third of a group of surgeons and oncologists reported finding out directly from their dying patients, their level of prognostic understanding , but only 2% had asked them directly (Fielding, Ko and Wong, 1995). Another study found that even when 86% of patients were judged to be competent, only 19% had been asked at some time before their resuscitation, of their wishes to be resuscitated if cardiac arrest occurred. In 68% of cases, physicians 'thought they knew what the patient wanted'. These same doctors acknowledged not having explored the topic with the patient (Bedell and Delbanco, 1984). The issues are not quite as simple as they appear. Before making such decisions, it is necessary to consider what the patient's perceived quality of life would be. Perceived quality of life is an important contributor to patient decisions about resuscitation (Starr, Perlman and Uhlmann, 1986; Zweibel, 1988).

It is also undeniably tricky to ask a patient, who is in hospital for surgery to replace a hip joint, if he or she wants to be resuscitated in the event of a cardiac arrest! Decisions about resuscitation are important and can be sources of stress themselves for nurses when carried out in an off-hand manner (Candy, 1991). (See the applications of the ADA model in Chapters 9 to 11 for how to avoid this dilemma.)

Maguire (1985) has described staff use of distancing tactics when faced with dying patients. An example is to perceive 'common' responses e.g. crying, in response to admission to an oncology ward as 'normal', rather than discussing with patients the causes for their upset and hence respecting their individuality. False reassurance and selectivity of attention on non-psychological aspects of care were other examples of distancing techniques. These strategies are used, according to Maguire, to protect both patient and staff from emotional over-exposure — preventing the patient from being excessively upset, and staff from 'burnout'. This is common in response to high demand situations where positive aspects are absent, e.g. intensive care nursing (Price and Bergen, 1977).

Multidisciplinary care with regular team meetings serve to keep all participants informed and to plan the management of individual patients. These teams can serve as a major source of support or stress for staff. If the team is driven by a leader who hands down pre-emptive decisions about care, then high levels of stress can result. A team where each member is encouraged to participate and where decisions about care are made after all members and the patient are consulted is much more likely to be a source of support for the staff.

Caring for the dying can be difficult, particularly for nurses who spend more time with the patient. The other health workers can leave the unit for respite, but not the nurse. General hospital care can be organized so that a supportive multidisciplinary team develops. But often, the least senior and experienced member of the medical team is left to make the most important decisions (Candy, 1991). Rivalry between teams and professional pride prevents cooperation and promotes competitive attitudes instead. Nurses are often caught between problems such as these rivalries and the demands of looking after the patient (High, 1989).

Nurses find it particularly stressful to deal with those patients who suffer intractable pain, who have young children, or who are afraid to die. In addition, dealing with psychiatric symptoms and with relatives are major sources of stress (Field, 1989; Alexander and Richie, 1990). Generally, those symptoms and situations which leave nurses feeling helpless and useless are the most stressful (Alexander and Ritchie, 1990).

It is hardly surprising, therefore, that nurses have developed psychological approaches for dealing with the stress of dying care. Most nurses are female and females may have a greater anxiety about death than male health workers (Ungar, Florian and Zernitski-Shurka, 1990), which may contribute to the difficulties many nurses face in caring for the dying. Nurses use a wide range of avoidance strategies with dying patients (Glaser and Strauss, 1965; Martin, 1983; Maguire, 1985).

Avoidance strategies limit opportunities for patients to gather information about their diagnosis and prognosis. The result is that there are differing levels of awareness of dying among patients in hospital, and these differences can be a source of tension. Glaser and Strauss (1965) described four levels of patient awareness of dying which have strong implications for communications:

1. Closed awareness: staff know, but the patient does not know that death is approaching.
2. Suspected awareness: staff know and the patient suspects he or she is dying and makes efforts to find out from the staff.
3. Mutual Pretence awareness: staff and patient know that death is approaching but there is an unspoken collusion between both parties not to acknowledge or discuss this.
4. Open awareness: staff and patient know and acknowledge that death is approaching and are prepared to discuss the issues.

In communications with the dying, staff should then:

1. Feel comfortable with the idea of mortality as normal, remembering,
   - that adaptation to the prospect of dying takes time
   - that the adaptation may not be smooth, in one direction, or consistent
   - that involvement of relatives helps all adapt better
   - that emotional upset is appropriate
   - but that upset may not always be seen
2. Arrange to make time available to the dying person in order to be with them, for discussion, or sometimes just to provide company to avoid the person feeling alone or not desired.
3. Establish from discussion with the patients, their desires for levels of treatment under what conditions, and develop multidisciplinary care plans based on this information.
4. Treat each patient as an individual and take care to avoid the use of distancing tactics.
5. Provide support for staff to minimize stress responses such as 'burnout'.

Relatives and patients, patients and relatives

> A man's dying is more the survivors' affair than his own.
>   Thomas Mann (1924)

Communications between the dying and their relatives facilitates the adaptation of both parties. Communication can help to resolve disputes within families and facilitates the adjustment of the relatives after the death of the patient (Parkes, 1972). Encouraging relatives to take as much part in the care of the patient as possible provides greater opportunities for the family to adapt to the process of a family member dying. It can also maintain the patient's sense of belonging for longer than might otherwise be the case.

However, communications can become 'blocked' within families if one or more members are unable to accept the patient's condition. There may be a silent agreement to avoid talking about anything to do with the patient's illness (Hinton, 1967). The community nurse, health visitor or family physician play key roles in caring for dying patients at home and attention must be given to patients' communication needs. This can be done while assisting in the physical care of the patient. These health workers can also aid the psychological care of the family by talking with family to identify problems, and helping the family resolve these.

Dying is a family affair, the death of one family member 'brings instantly into being a whole new network of relations between you and the ideas, the desires, the habits of the (family member) now dead. It is a re-arrangement of the world' (D'Saint-Exupery, 1942). Involvement of the family should be encouraged as an important part of the adaptation process for all concerned, particularly for dying children. Involvement of siblings in the care of a dying child can be beneficial to both parties, and may help assuage some of the feelings of guilt often felt by the surviving siblings (Wass, 1984).

Open communication versus mutual pretence

Glaser and Strauss's (1965) state of open awareness translates to an open communication condition: when all those involved in the care of the dying patient — particularly the patient — recognize, acknowledge and are willing to talk about issues surrounding the patient's impending death. Mutual pretence refers to the state of affairs where all those involved, including the patient, all know the patient is dying, but no acknowledgment of this is made. Hence pretence that all is well is required. This creates strain for all involved, often leading to social death. It also requires participants to turn a blind eye to the often obvious signs of anxiety and sadness, and makes honest communication of feelings almost impossible. This can be particularly hard for dying children (Wass, 1984; Waechter, 1987).

Spending time

Adaptation is most likely if the patient and close relatives spend time together (Hinton, 1967; Parkes, 1972). Spending time is important for several reasons. It is also valuable for relatives to be able to spend time with dying patients, perhaps doing things for them, perhaps just being with them, helping them to feel that they have had the most of the remaining time with their family. Anticipatory grieving can and does occur together (Hinton, 1967). Sweeting and Gilhooly (1990) identified six adaptation tasks for the patient and family to deal with:

1. Remain involved with the patient — responding to the patient's experience and share the experience of the rest of the family.
2. Remain separate from the patient — believing in oneself as an individual who can and will exist in a future without the patient.
3. Adapt suitably to role changes — assuming immediate new duties and anticipating future new responsibilities.
4. Bear the affects of grief — acknowledging and expressing the feelings aroused by terminal illness.
5. Come to terms with the reality of impending loss — being able to tolerate thoughts of the future and making practical plans required to deal with it.
6. Say goodbye — acknowledging the end is near and communicating a verbal or non-verbal farewell.

It is also important for staff to be prepared to spend time with patients whose family can't or won't spend time with them, or who have no close family. In this case, staff provide the human warmth that presence of another caring person can bring. Talking, reading to the patient or even listening to music, or watching TV can all be valuable. What is important is the quality of time spent and the attitude of the staff.

The importance of empathic understanding

At few other times in a person's life is there likely to be such a potential sense of aloneness as during the dying phase. Sometimes, this makes itself felt in the presence of others. Sometimes, relatives will find they cannot easily cope, and patients may find they are giving support to their relative. Understanding can be greatly enhanced by empathy — the attempted sharing of each others' experiences.

The process of empathic understanding has been outlined in earlier chapters and so will not be dealt with in great depth here. (See chapters on handling emotions and breaking bad news for more discussion of empathic understanding.)

Dying children

> What greater pain could mortals have than this:
> to see their children dead before their eyes?
>
> Euripides (c.421 BC)

Most childhood deaths in industrialized countries occur either during or shortly after birth, from obstetric complications, or more rarely within the first year of life. In older children death from accident is the most common cause. Chronic disease is mostly responsible for other deaths, with malignancy being frequent. The most common malignancy in children is acute lymphoblastic leukemia; currently about 60% of children survive five years or longer from the time of diagnosis (Van Eys, 1981). It has been argued that for childhood cancers there is a vital need for the assumption that cure is possible (Van Eys, 1981), and it might be argued that this could equally apply to other conditions, such as chronic renal failure and certain other fatal systemic diseases of childhood. It is important for the whole family to retain hope and belief in the possibility of cure. The age of the child is influential in understanding the need for hospitalization and treatment, and determines available coping skills (see Chapter 3). The low infant and child mortality in developed countries is a fairly recent phenomenon but most parents have not seen an adult die, let alone a child. In many developing countries, death of children is, if not expected, then perhaps more readily acknowledged as the (avoidable) norm (Videka-Sherman,1982). It should not, however, be assumed to be any less painful.

Younger children seem to be able to accept the idea of dying at least as well as adults (Lamerton, 1973; Jeffrey and Lansdown, 1982). Though their understanding of death may be less than that of adults, children aged above three years have growing conceptions of death. An understanding of the irreversibility, non-functionality and universality of death occurs between five to seven years of age (Speece and Brent, 1988). The concept of death seems to be fully formed by nine years of age (Anthony, 1972; Kastenbaum, 1974; Kane, 1979).

The principles of keeping patients informed of their condition apply to both adults and children. The child has to live with the consequences of decisions (Shield and Baum, 1994). The major difference is in how to communicate with children. Children's developmental level influences their concept of disease and death, influencing comprehension of the need for treatment. Therefore, communications must be at a level appropriate for the developmental level of the child and should aim at helping the child understand, irrespective of age. This is an important example of the principle that all communications with patients should be made in terms that they are likely to understand.

Younger children, aged six months or over, will often have more anxiety about being separated from their families (Lamerton, 1973), about fear of death of another child in hospital (Natterson and Knudson, 1960), and about painful medical procedures than about dying (Lamerton, 1973; Waechter, 1988). It has been reported that younger children will sometimes reject their parents for not protecting them from the painful medical procedures they may undergo (Friedman, Chodoff and Mason, 1963).

Children from six or seven years onward may have unexpected anxieties, not about dying but about treatments, especially those which are mutilative (Knudson and Natterson, 1960; Alderson, 1993). The anxieties extend to the extent that they will be 'different' from other children. Normalcy should be maintained when and where possible for all children, especially in attending school, continuing to interact with peers, etc. (Jeffrey and Landsdown, 1982). Withdrawal during acute stages of illness often occurs (Woon, 1983), and desire for privacy and time alone should be permitted wherever possible. Teenagers would normally spend time alone from the family, and it is important to remember that children still have their normal developmental needs, in spite of their illness. The more special kindness shown to a dying child, however, the more worried the child may become if the child has not been informed and if adults are unwilling to discuss the illness (Bluebond-Langner, 1978).

Honesty is thus very important with children and teenagers. Young people are much less forgiving of abuses of trust. Loss of trust may cause many problems for the team trying to provide care for the family. This is an important point. In caring for dying children, health workers must maintain awareness that the family, and not just the child, should be considered. The stresses on parents and siblings of dying children can be enormous (Videka-Sherman,1982; Balk, 1983). It has been reported that dying children seldom ask direct questions on the topic of their own death, seemingly to protect their parents, and mutual pretence seems to predominate within the family (Bluebond-Langner, 1978). The psychological cost of this to the dying child is not clear, but it is likely to be high.

It is much more difficult to provide effective care for a child whose family is unable to cope with the implications of the child's illness. The health worker should anticipate that the child may feel responsible and guilty of causing suffering in beloved family members. If this occurs, the child and family need counselling to deal with this. Depression may occur in response to pain and as anticipatory loss.

Psychotherapists have long argued that children are prone to perceive illness as a punishment for past angry wishes (Perrin and Gerrity, 1981). It has been suggested that siblings may also believe they are somehow responsible for the illness of their brother or sister because of earlier wishes arising out of sibling rivalry and other common developmental ambivalence. Siblings may be pushed out by the focus on the patient and the parents. The siblings may be very much in need of help in adapting to the loss of a brother or sister (Wass, 1984). It is important in communications with children generally to explain fully that their disease is not some kind of punishment for past thoughts and wishes.

Communications strategies with children should then:

1. Be broadly the same as those adopted with adults:
   * honest
   * informative
   * at a level appropriate to the child's developmental age
   * explore the child's illness representations and causal attributions
2. Include at least parents and siblings, if not other family members.
3. Maintain as positive an attitude to recovery as possible, without resorting to telling lies if prognosis is bleak.
4. Provide care within the framework of the child's family, wherever and whenever feasible.
5. Retain normalcy and recognize and respect the child's normal developmental needs. Having fun, laughter, birthday and other parties is particularly important.

Communicating with the bereaved

> One cannot live with the dead;
> Either we die with them,
> Or we make them live again.
> Or we forget them.
>
> Martin-Chauffier (1947)

Bereavement brings the need for adaptation. This takes time and is by definition painful. Grief, which characterizes bereavement, is the process of giving up the feelings invested in the lost person. Certain features of adjustment to loss may be identified as characteristic of the human loss response. These include elements of:

* initial denial/shock, especially where death is unexpected, e.g. following road accidents
* arousal, agitation, searching behaviour broadly comparable to a need to find the lost person

- acute 'pangs' of grief, where the loss of the person is acutely felt, featuring deep psychological pain, accompanied by crying, and often calling the name of the lost person
- 'finding' behaviour in the absence of the lost person, e.g. dreaming, hallucinating and other perceptual phenomena, sometimes called mitigation behaviour
- detachment
- eventual adaptation (Parkes, 1978)

This process can take many months, and apparently cannot be hurried (Parkes, 1978). Often years may pass before the bereaved person becomes adapted to the loss. An acute sense of loss may re-emerge after many years, such as on anniversaries, or at significant times, such as at offspring's weddings. Grieving is normal and appropriate behaviour in the face of loss and is necessary if detachment from the lost person and subsequent adaptation to the loss are to occur (Parkes, 1978). Failure to detach and adapt can lead to chronic problems for the bereaved. This pathological grief reaction is indicated by continued and unusually prolonged grief, failure to acknowledge the reality of the loss, depression, and/or interference with normal function, and requires psychotherapeutic treatment.

An impressive number of studies have shown the recently bereaved to be at greater risk of morbidity and mortality from all kinds of minor and major illness (Parkes, 1978). Health workers should be aware of this and make arrangements to monitor the health of the bereaved person if necessary, especially in the care of the elderly spouse who is left alone by bereavement.

In communicating with the bereaved, then, the following points should be considered:
- Grief should *not* be discouraged or suppressed.
- Restlessness, anxiety and pangs of grief seem to be necessary to adapt to loss. Support and empathic understanding can be helpful.
- Explanation of the role of grieving and the time it can take before adjustment occurs need to be made.
- At subsequent contact, consider exploring the bereaved's health.
- Be prepared to discuss the dead person with the bereaved. Changing the subject is often a distancing tactic.
- Anticipatory grief may appear both in relatives and a dying patient before death occurs. This is normal.
- Follow up, or arrange for others to, the bereaved family.

It is important that death be handled sensitively and openly in hospitals. Failure to do this can result in disillusionment with health services and costly litigation (Hughes and Henley, 1990).

▇▇ Communication technique

Identifying information needs

Communication technique with the dying involves a preparatory phase, where information should be obtained on the patient's desire for information and participatory involvement. This may be formalized as part of an initial or admission interview, or informal. Use the ADA approach (see Chapters 9–11).

Maintain optimism

Find something positive to say to the patient. Remember, retaining hope is important in coping with treatment and adaptation. Some workers place heavy emphasis on the importance of 'sincere, controlled optimism' (Brewin, 1991). Optimism is associated with more positive health outcomes and lower levels of handicap. Optimistic patients may live longer than pessimistic patients. Optimism among staff reduces the demand placed on staff and may help prevent depression among patients. However, inappropriate optimism in the patient may indicate an inability to accept deterioration; that among staff may be a risk factor for burnout (see Chapter 13). There is always something that can be done for dying patients, even if it is simply sitting with them until they are asleep, for example. In care of dying people, such acts must count as having equal priority along with other more traditional care tasks (Herth, 1990).

Handling uncertainty

A major difficulty faced by patients, relatives and health workers involves uncertainty. Handling the uncertainty of dying in a way that helps maintain a positive and desirable outlook can be difficult. Maguire and Faulkner (1988) suggested the health worker should explain the uncertainty, identify if it is a problem for the patient/relative, and give information the person may use to better understand the progress of the illness (e.g. signs of treatment versus deterioration).

Maintaining close contact between the health worker and patient also helps minimize uncertainty. Frequent discussion with the patient/relative provides information, helps with planning visits and reassures the patient/relative. Fewer unforeseen developments then occur. The health worker maintains a supportive relationship for the family, which will increase their available resources and help them cope better. The example is loosely modelled on Maguire and Faulkner (1988).

HW: I expect that this uncertainty is quite difficult for you to cope with, is it?

Pt/R: Yes. I don't know what to do, whether to make plans or just wait for, you know .., the end. Each time I feel tired, I think, is this it?

HW: I wish I could be less unsure about the progress of your illness. It sounds like the uncertainty is quite a strain for you.

Pt/R: It is.

HW: Would it help if I told you what sorts of signs to look out for, that might indicate that the condition is deteriorating? If you don't want to know, I won't tell you.

Pt/R: I think it would help, even if it only tells me when not to think the worst.

HW: Okay, well, I expect that there will be more weakness than usual and that your appetite will be worse first. Would you like to know more?

Pt/R: Sometimes weakness is a problem now.

HW: Yes. But you can expect it to become worse quite quickly if the condition deteriorates, perhaps over one or two days, and there will be less energy to get up and move around. Once this stage is reached, and if you'd like me to, I will tell you more if you like. Does that sound okay?

Pt/R: Yes, that sounds fine.

Use reflective questions to explore the worries the patient may have, to recognize the causes of concern for patients/relatives. This enables clear identification of problem areas for the patient/relative, many of which might be easily dealt with.

Collusion

Collusion is also a common problem faced by relatives and patients, and health workers often join in to maintain a mutual pretence that all is well. Collusion is an unspoken conspiracy to maintain a mutual pretence in this case. Again, Maguire and Faulkner (1988) made valuable suggestions about an approach towards dealing with collusion. They suggest asking one of the two (or more) colluding parties (usually a patient and close relative, such as spouse) for permission to check if the second person is aware of the situation to the same extent as the first.

In other words, the task of the health professional is to act as arbitrator between the two persons, to identify if both parties know the gravity of the situation, and if so, encourage them to agree to opening up their understanding to include the partner's knowledge. This results in release of unnecessary stress caused by maintaining the pretence that all is well, when it is not. The advantage of disclosure of bad news initially to both parties simultaneously helps minimize the development of collusion, but is not guaranteed to prevent it developing subsequently.

What happens if one party does not agree to the other person being informed? One strategy is to tell the relative that the patient is the health worker's first responsibility if the patient wants information then it will be given. Maguire and Faulkner (1988) suggest a slightly less confronta-tional approach:

HW: I've spoken with your husband and he doesn't fully realize the seriousness of his condition. He really ought to be informed as he was asking for more information. The only reason I didn't tell him was because I promised you I wouldn't, but I think we need to reconsider this.

R: No. I don't want to see him hurt. I don't think he could cope with this.

HW: Well, you know him better than I do, but it would help if you told me why you think he would not be able to cope with the news.

R: Yes. He wants to go to Australia for a holiday next summer. Our son lives there, and he's been saving up, looking forward to going so much. I couldn't stand to see him so disappointed.

HW: I see. Is there any other reason?

R: I just think he'd give up, not try any more, and then . . .

HW: Then what?

R: Then he'll . . . go so much sooner.

HW: Any other reasons?

R: No.

HW: Okay. Well, I can understand you're not wanting to tell him, but there might be other ways of resolving this.

R: How?

HW: I will talk with him. I do not intend to tell him, but it might be that he already suspects a lot more than you think he does. He might reveal that he knows he has cancer, then there wouldn't be any point in maintaining the pretence.

R: Well, if you promise not to tell him.

HW: I won't tell him, but if he knows his situation and asks me to confirm it, then I must.

In this situation, Maguire and Faulkner (1988) recommend that, if the patient does strongly suspect, then they should have their suspicions con-firmed by the health worker. Then, you should seek the patient's permission to inform the relative of his knowledge.

Once all parties are aware that pretence is no longer necessary, there may be more expression of emotion, some directed at the health workers from time to time. This may be difficult for the health worker, but there may be opportunities for giving further help. The health worker can avoid taking things personally.

Other communications with dying patients should be handled in as normal a way as possible, and should not need special mention.

Techniques useful in communication with children

Parental involvement should be considered a priority, and can be therapeutic for all involved. Children are usually able to talk naturally about death; those under six years of age may show little fear of dying though more about separation and treatment. Increasing the child's control over pain, especially that associated with medical or nursing procedures, is important. Communications which inform the child about procedures, and those which give information on sensory experience during the procedure are both important components (see Chapter 9).

Inaccurate perceptions of the reasons for hospitalization and the causes of illness should be explored and corrected, otherwise these can be major sources of anxiety. With children less than about six years old, drawing is useful to explore the child's feelings. Imagery may also be used to good effect in other ways (LeBaron and Zeltzer, 1985).

A ten-year-old or adolescent might be able to deal with a question such as: 'Why do you think this has happened to you?' But younger children may have difficulty. Direct answers to a question of this type will be the exception. Instead, use empathic statements as these can be powerful in building up conversations with young children:

> If I was a little boy who had to come into hospital with an illness like yours, I might wonder why this was happening to me. Is that how you feel?

However, be careful not to put ideas into the child's head! The example of other children can also be helpful in indicating to the child that the nurse providing the care understands the way they feel.

> I talked to one little girl in here who thought she got sick because of something she did wrong. Do you ever feel like that?

Hospitalization makes young children feel they are being punished. They may plead with their parents and staff and the next moment rage helplessly against those looking after them for allowing these things to happen (Wass, 1984). It becomes important to accept the child's expressions of anger uncritically. Explanation to the parents of the ambivalence the child might be experiencing can help adults cope with their child. The best policy is to keep the child at home with the family whenever and wherever possible, and maintain close contact with the family.

Wass (1984) suggests explaining cause and effect relationships between disease, hospitalization and treatment, even where the child does not understand. The purpose of this is somewhat obscure, when with a little forethought and sensitivity, an explanation can usually be made in a way the child is likely to understand.

> You know your blood is very tired? Well, we have to give your blood some medicine to help it work better. But the only way I can give you this medicine is through a little tube into your arm. Do you think that would be OK? If I'm going to do this, you have to come into the hospital, because that's where we do these sorts of things. There are lots of doctors and nurses there to look after people, and other children to play with.

Technical accuracy in the explanation is probably less important than achieving some level of comprehension. Nonetheless, explanations should always be given, even if understanding is not achieved. What is important is that the children feel they can understand why these things happen. Young patients should be given control over aspects of their care. To achieve this they must be given permission and often encouragment to participate by exercising control wherever this is practical. Lewis, Lewis, Lorrimer and Palmer (1977) state, ' . . . until we accept the fact that each future adult must be responsible for his own health and treat him accordingly, we shall always be looking to others for that which can only come from within'. This should be at least choice of nurse, choice of site of injection, encouraging to help by participating in the care in little ways, and informed consent for surgery (Shield and Baum, 1994). Repetition of simple explanations for what is happening to the child is one way of involving parents.

Emphasize that the child is not to blame for what is happening; that it is not the child's fault; that the child is not being punished; that sometimes helping the child can be uncomfortable for the child, but is needed to get the child well again, and so on. Reiterate these points frequently and in various ways.

Use of a caring and gentle voice, touch, and spending time with sick children, valuing them and their work all help to counteract the perception that they are bad and being punished.

Normal rules and regulations about appropriate behaviour should be retained despite the child's illness or parental guilt. These rules provide security and consistency for the child and helps to contribute to an established normalcy. These rules should of course be applied in a warm and positive manner, ideally in the same way they have always been applied. Avoid a cold and punitive manner.

For older children of school age or middle-childhood, their more sophisticated language skills enable them to articulate thoughts, fears and other feelings, and to understand simple cause of illness and the need for treatment. Explanation is a high priority, as is the need to maintain control. This means giving lots of information, consulting the children, and giving them as many opportunities to exercise choice as possible.

School-aged children may have many questions about death that may seem morbid to some adults. They are reportedly very pre-occupied with the details of death and decay, and life after death (Wass, 1984; Waechter, 1988). Parental openness to dialogue with the child should be encouraged (Waechter, 1988). These questions should be answered but succinctly and neutrally.

Some children, like some adults, prefer not to face the truth and try hard to retain a pretence that all is well. This wish not to confront the dying should be respected while it lasts. Most children eventually seem to realize and confront the truth (Wass, 1984). School-aged children need to feel able to express their emotions and parents should ideally share these and provide support at such times.

> I expect it must be quite scary not knowing what's going to happen next?
> If you feel like shouting, you do that. Shouting can help a lot sometimes when you feel all tight inside.
> Its a good thing to cry and we all need to do it from time to time.
> You look very sad today. Can I give you a hug?
> Would you like to have some fun today? What would you like to do?

Adolescents may feel a greater sense of bitterness and anger over their situation. They may need to talk more to come to terms with their experience. Contact with peers, though important for all hospitalized children, is particularly important in older children and adolescents.

Appearances are an important aspect of communication. For older children and adolescents, being acceptable to their friends is a very important developmental need. Effort should be made to help young patients appear to others as they want, not only when visitors are expected, but at all other times.

Parents in particular may be the target of adolescent anger and communications should be directed at explaining that this is not abnormal. Parents should be supported and encouraged not to retaliate. Emphasizing the normal developmental needs of a young patient and pointing out how these needs are thwarted by disease can help parents or new staff better understand the powerful feelings that might be displayed.

Techniques in communication with bereaved parents

Many of the approaches to breaking news to the bereaved have already been outlined in Chapter 11. The following deals with one important aspect of death telling — breaking news of a child's death to the parents.

If breaking the news of a death is one of the most demanding aspects of a health worker's job, informing parents of the death of their child must be among the most difficult situations. Few studies have explored this aspect of health care. A recently published report found one in three bereaved couples felt the interview informing them of the death of their child was either badly handled or offensive. Police were rated as more sympathetic than nurses, but the former receive special training on how to do this. Finlay and Dallimore (1991) found little evidence that breaking this news is handled any better today than 10 years ago.

Parents reported that reasonable or sympathetic informants had an understanding and caring attitude, did not hurry the parents, answered questions, checked that the parents understood the news, and designated a person whom they could subsequently consult for further information. By contrast, parents who met with evasive responses, or where questions were unanswered 'felt that a cover-up had occurred' (Finlay and Dallimore, 1991).

Eighty-one of 109 parents had seen their child's body after death (irrespective of cause of death, which included road and other accident, medical problems, suicide and murder). Only the mother of a murdered girl reportedly regretted this. Forty-nine felt they had had insufficient time with the body, especially if death was due to road accident. Twenty-eight parents did not see the body and subsequently deeply regretted this. Several parents expressed deep regret that they were not able to hold, lay out, wash or even touch their child's body (Finlay and Dallimore, 1991).

Only 16 parents had a follow-up contact from anyone at the hospital after the death. In three cases, this was from a transplant coordinator. Few parents thought they were shown any care at hospital immediately after the child's death. Some parents were kept waiting up to three-and-a-half hours without any information on the resuscitation attempts being made on their child (Finlay and Dallimore, 1991).

Communications in this special case of death telling should include:
- meeting the parents in private
- providing the information in an unhurried manner
- showing respect for the parents and the enormity of their loss
- showing a caring and understanding attitude
- allowing parents time to ask questions as they arise
- answering such questions openly and honestly
- checking to ensure that the parents understand the news
- encouraging to the parents to spend as much time as they wish with their dead child
- providing a private place where they may be together with their child in an unhurried way
- taking the time and trouble to contact the parents subsequent to the death, on a number of occasions over the ensuing period

The following example illustrates how a parent who has just reached the hospital might be informed of the death by accidental drowning of their child.

Parent: How is he? Is he all right? I want to see him!

HW: I'll take you to see him in moment, but I need to tell you something first.

Parent: What, what's wrong?

HW: Peter had been in the water a long time. By the time the ambulance team reached him, his heart had stopped beating.

Parent: Oh no, this isn't happening!

HW: The ambulance team worked on him all the way from the lake. We did also. We've spent almost two hours trying to re-start his heart. We weren't able to. I'm sorry.

Parent: I don't believe you. He can't be. He was. . . that policeman said he'd only been in the water a few minutes! That's not . . . (breaks down crying).

(Long pause.)

HW: Your husband should be here any moment now. I think it best that you wait for him before seeing Peter. It would be better for both of you.

Such communications *should not* be given by a person who is
- cold and businesslike
- lacking in good interpersonal skills
- lacking in empathy

- hurried
- delayed
- dismissive or evasive of questions
- unwilling to allow parents time to ask question or be with their child

There is a substantial literature now available on effective care of the dying person. This chapter has covered some of the aspects felt to be important. It is by no means exhaustive. It has focused on those areas in which communications are important. As you will have seen, care is intrinsically the communication of concern and acceptance.

Exercises

As with previous role-play exercises, these may be most effective if individuals (other members of the department or other departments, students, or actors) can play the role of the patient. It is likely to make the exercise more realistic. If this is not feasible, then turn taking or allocation to specific roles is recommended.

Because of the nature of these role-plays, it is advisable to spend some time discussing the participants' feelings about the roles. Sometimes, participants can closely identify with a particular role and may find it disturbing. Thus, carrying out a de-briefing after the completion of the exercise is important.

1. *You are the patient.* (Be your self as much as possible.) Six months ago, you were diagnosed as having leukemia. At the time, you were given extensive treatment, including anti-cancer chemotherapy which made you feel very, very ill. The treatment did help to slow the progress of the disease. Recently, you have felt weak once more, and your doctor told you you had a recurrence of the disease. You finished a second course of anti-cancer treatment two weeks ago, but it has not slowed the disease this time. The doctor has told you that it is unlikely the leukemia can be controlled this time. The doctor has suggested you have a course of whole-body irradiation, bone marrow transplantation, and repeat stronger chemotherapy. Even then, it may not help. The last treatment you had made you feel so bad, you do not feel you can face it more.

   You have decided to say no to further treatment and have

asked to see your health professional to announce your decision.

You are the health professional.   Your patient is the participant's own age and background. Six months ago the patient was diagnosed as having leukemia, which responded sluggishly to a moderate anti-cancer chemotherapy programme, but the disease 'stalled' and did not progress further. About two months ago, deterioration of the condition occurred with the patient reporting greater fatigue. The patient was told that whole-body irradiation and bone marrow transplantation was needed. This should halt the disease, but the probability of this is somewhat uncertain. Treatment would be very unpleasant for the patient. The doctor who has been caring for this patient in the past is no longer working at your establishment. The patient has asked to see you.

Task: To discuss the treatment options and decide on treatment.
Time available: 20 minutes.

2.   *You are the patient.*   (Be yourself as much as possible.) Two years ago, while travelling abroad, you were involved in a road accident, and because of a femoral arterial laceration, you lost a lot of blood. You were given a transfusion of packed cells and Ringer's lactate. You recovered well.

   These last few months you have been under a lot of stress at work and outside of work. About one month ago, you developed a high fever following a chest infection and your doctor diagnosed pneumonia. You spent eight days in hospital, given antibiotics and recovered well, though you have remained tired. While in hospital, your doctor told you that they wanted to do some blood tests. You agreed. A few days later, your doctor told you that the test needed to be repeated. Those results, so your doctor said, showed you to have both antibodies to HIV and to have an abnormal white blood cell pattern. The physician tells you this means you have an HIV-related syndrome.

   You feel very scared and very confused. You do not know how you have caught this virus, and though you are well at present, the chance of further recurrence is very high. You do not know either if you will get sick and die, or if you will remain well. You feel very angry and bitter and have lost all desire to work, or to interact with your family. You feel embarrassed and are ashamed in case your work colleagues find out and treat you like an invalid or worse. You are also scared. Mostly you feel like you have been cheated. You find yourself asking the questions 'How have I got this?' and 'What have I done to deserve this?' You find yourself unable to get out of this state.

You are the health worker. Your patient has recently been diagnosed as HIV positive and one month ago showed signs of an opportunistic pneumonia which was successfully treated. The patient has AIDS-related syndrome. At present the patient's condition is stable, but could deteriorate at any time. You were asked to call and see the patient who is they are reported to be 'depressed'.

Task: to identify the main concerns of the patient and to help them work towards a state where the patient can more effectively function.
Time available: 20 minutes.

3. *You are the patient.* (Be yourself as much as possible.) Three months ago you were taken ill and admitted to hospital after collapsing at work. At the time you were diagnosed as having pneumonia, but tests showed you had a viral infection of the heart. You have increasingly been unable to move very much on your own. You feel tired and breathless most of the time. At the time of diagnosis, the doctor did not tell you very much about how long you would be ill for. You have noticed that you are not getting any stronger, and some days it is difficult to get out of bed. You feel very frightened and worry about recovering from the illness. Your family has been trying to cheer you up, but they are obviously all very unhappy and very worried. They particularly keep talking about when you are 'back on your feet again'. You do not want to discuss this with your family because you don't want to upset them, but you are afraid you might be dying.
      You want to discuss the illness with your health worker.

You are the health worker. Three months ago your patient collapsed following the onset of a viral infection of the heart, which has lead to a progressive cardiomyopathy, or deterioration of the heart muscle. This profoundly weakens the muscle of the heart so much that the patient is physically disabled. The condition is progressive and the patient is dying. There is no effective treatment, other than palliative care and symptomatic treatment. The relatives have discussed with you that the patient does not know the diagnosis, but appears to be anxious and depressed. The family are supportive and caring about the patient, but are finding the situation very difficult.

Task: to identify the patient's problems and come up with a resolution.
Time available: 20 minutes.

Discussion

1. Though it occurs rarely, suicide can be a choice made by some people with a terminal illness. What do you think are the important determinants of a choice to commit suicide, and what would your role be if the patient implied to you an intention to commit suicide or asked you for assistance?

2. How much should patients in the terminal stages of their lives be encouraged to take responsibility for decisions regarding their treatment, assuming they have the mental capacity to do so?

3. How much autonomy should children be encouraged to take when terminally ill, and how much should health professionals be guided by those wishes where they contradict the preferences of the health workers or their parents? At what age should autonomy be respected?

4. If an adolescent patient with serious, painful condition, which is not immediately fatal but will kill the patient within 12 months, expressly requests you not to provide treatment, and the parents have urged you to do what you can to treat their child, what should you do? What would you do? Why?

13

Communications With Other Health Workers and Related Issues

Educational Objectives

By the end of this chapter , you should be able to

- recognize and describe two classes of communication important to individuals within an organization
- discuss the relationship of the individual to the organization
- specify the importance of a positive attitude in good interprofessional communication
- cite the hazards associated with poor inter- and intra-professional communications
- explain the importance of factors such as role expectations and professional hierarchies as obstacles to good staff communications
- explain at least eight barriers to good staff communications
- explain and apply a simple three-point plan of implementing change in unit communications
- identify and discuss at least ten ways of facilitating staff communications
- explain the communications advantages in adopting collaborative styles of practice
- discuss the application of feedback and empathy in staff communications
- differentiate and define evaluation and feedback
- outline the main requirements of written care/medical records
- plan being interviewed by the media
- specify and demonstrate the main features of providing staff support

Introduction

All organizations need communications to function. Without this they grind to a halt almost instantly. Health care organizations are highly complex and are particularly dependent on communication within and between clinical, managerial and administrative levels. Each professional group's own management hierarchy has to function efficiently, and the organizational administration has to be able to provide the necessary resources needed for the professionals to provide appropriate levels of input. On the clinical level, different medical, nursing and allied health professionals have to integrate their skills to provide high levels of care. A further role involves developing a health services organization through the introduction of new areas of service (e.g. adolescent health), new styles of working (e.g. primary nursing) and individual staff training.

The health care organization usually succeeds in providing health care, but at considerable costs in terms of efficiency, staff burnout, low staff morale, strained managerial relations, litigation and administrative unresponsiveness. Ultimately, it is patient care that suffers. Most health professionals genuinely try to do their best for patients, yet may recognize that less that optimal service is provided. Feelings of frustration are understandably common (Ward, Peat and Revill, 1994). Reasons for this are explored more thoroughly below.

Not surprisingly, the reasons include the same kinds of attitudes we encountered in exploring problems of information-giving to patients — beliefs that someone else has given the information; that others don't want or need to know; and insufficient time. In addition, traditional organizational problems of communication are overlaid on these, including top-down information flow; entrenched attitudes about roles in the face of changes; and inaccurate beliefs about who knows what. These factors when coupled with certain task demands can reduce feelings of participation, predictability and control, thereby affecting job satisfaction, and ultimately staff health.

There are many examples of poor communication between different health professionals (Walton and McLachlan, 1986) and between different levels of the management hierarchy (Bauby, 1972; Hamilton, 1987). This chapter focuses on communications between health workers and suggests methods for communications with the media and other non-patient/relative groups encountered in health care. The use of different barriers and facilitators to improved communication, both written and verbal, are explored and suggestions made for overcoming these.

The individual within an organization

Within any group, an individual needs to feel valued both as a worker and as a person. From these two factors, most people derive their sense of self-esteem. (Though other factors are involved in self-respect, these are the most important in the work context.) Maslow (1954) proposed a hierarchy of individual needs which he argued were important in understanding why people work and what they communicate about. The five levels of Maslow's hierarchy are:

Need for self-actualization and autonomous self-respect
Need for respect and esteem from peers
Need for a sense of belonging, companionship and love
Need for safety and security
Need for food and shelter

The main feature of Maslow's model is that lower needs must be satisfied before higher needs are addressed. In other words, someone who has not eaten for one week and is homeless is not going to be concerned too much with autonomous self-respect; there is a greater need to look for food and shelter. Similarly, a person who has no respect from peers and has no sense of belonging and companionship is unlikely to achieve self-actualizing and self-respect. These needs determine motivation. That is, Maslow argued, innate needs motivate a person to seek the fulfilment of those needs.

From Maslow's model, we can identify two broad overlapping areas of communication needs for health workers. (There are other areas but for our purposes we will focus on just these two.) These will be called task-oriented and performance-oriented communications. Task-oriented communications refer to verbal, non-verbal or written communications addressing the execution of the health worker's professional role. They include information about patient care tasks, general information about patients, shift-duty rotas, case notes, etc. Task-oriented communications also include information on care outcomes, feedback on a patient's condition and other evaluative data which may also carry information about performance. These aspects of task-oriented communication overlap with performance-oriented communications, which relate directly to the self, either the professional self (in the overlap from task-related communications), or the social self. This later category includes non-patient directed communications, such as relationship-building conversations and other communications where the primary purpose is social rather than task-oriented. A key component in social communications are evaluative responses. Evaluations, either professional or social, are judgemental in nature. Thus they have a moral component and say things about the worth of the person or the person's acts (which many people mistakenly perceive as synonymous). Evaluations may be explicit, as when a tutor or consultant comments on a job well done, or when a colleague evaluates our appearance with a critical comment. They may also be implicit, as when a unit manager is not consulted about proposed changes, or when a person is passed over for promotion.

In contrast to evaluations there are also performance/self communications called feedback. Feedback is evaluation without the judgement. It is a non-judgemental communication to another with the purpose of facilitating self-awareness. Feedback is a necessary component if improvement in performance is desired. Improvement occurs without feedback, provid the person sees a need to change and has the potential for change. However, more positive and consistent performance changes occur with accurate feedback. Self-awareness enables individuals to realize the consequences of their actions. They may then choose to repeat their actions if the consequences are favourable, or to modify their actions to produce more desirable results.

Evaluative judgements are usually based on specified or unspecified performance criteria. Where performance standards are explicit, the individuals can then compare their performance with the expected standard. In most cases, performance standards are not explicit, or standards or criteria considered important vary from person to person or place to place.

People can perform to standards when the standard is known and achievable within the structural limitations of the work environment. Structural limitations include staffing levels, role restrictions and managerial expectations. Stress is more likely when standards are not explicit, when they relate more to the evaluator's value system than specified or shared criteria, or when the limitations of the person's working environment prevent adequate performance, and the consequences of poor performance are severe and subsequently uncontrollable.

People experience stress when they perceive demands outweigh resources, and when there is an anticipated threat. The nature of the threat may be to the person's self-esteem, professional standing in the eyes of others, or perceived social acceptability. Maslow's model implies that where peer respect is absent, self-respect may be more difficult to achieve; where social acceptance is absent, so peer respect and self-respect are more likely to be absent.

Badly designed or maintained management hierarchies tend to rain communications down on the shop-floor workers from on high, and seldom move in the opposite direction. The system makes no allowance for the feelings or opinions of these same workers. The implicit message is 'your opinions don't count'. Workers feel undervalued, conflicts are not resolved, and dissatisfactions accumulate. These dissatisfactions do not reach the management in a positive way.

The only responses open to individuals are to be passively resistant to managerial wishes and avoid commitment to the organization. More often dissatisfaction is expressed through high sickness absenteeism or high staff turnover. Organizations that fail to accommodate the individual's communication needs show characteristic symptoms of communication problems (Bauby, 1976; Hamilton, 1987).

Common difficulties in professional communications

Doctors more than any other health care group are criticized for poor communications with other health care providers. This occurs in Europe (Walton and McLachlan, 1986) and the USA (Larkin 1988), and is probably so elsewhere. There seems to be a number of reasons for this. The first explanation is a lack of physician time. There are fewer doctors than nurses, and fewer physiotherapists, clinical psychologists, occupational therapists, dietitians, speech therapists, play-therapists, social workers, and other allied professional groups than doctors. The argument that there isn't the opportunity to meet with other care providers can only partly be sustained. Differences in the timing of nursing shifts, medical rounds and clinics may mean that there are times in the day when a particular doctor is less accessible. But then a doctor often has less time available to talk also. Thus, a chance meeting in a corridor, or a few minutes' conversation in the canteen may be the only chance health workers have to communicate.

One of the prime reasons identified by Ley (1977) as to why doctors did not give information to patients was lack of time. Yet when special efforts were made to communicate, patients were still dissatisfied. There seems to be a suspiciously similar parallel here.

Threats to professional integrity

Many members of the medical profession feel threatened by the developments in other professions and the increasingly apparent erosion of doctors' 'traditional' authority. Considerable evidence disputes the argument that in the past, all other professions were 'supplementary' to medicine. Indeed, some groups, such as midwives, apparently resisted to the last moment inviting a doctor's participation (Freeling, 1986). There is also a lack of understanding of the role requirements of other professional groups involved in health care (Freeling, 1986) and what skills other professional groups can actually provide in terms of health care. Many doctors have not realized that other professional groups have specialized to a variable extent as has their own profession. The introduction of concepts such as nursing diagnosis may seem particularly threatening. Others, such as multidisciplinary team care, may be seen in a different light by the doctor and everyone else. Where attitudes are not shared, shared understanding is rarer. Medical groups in some parts of the world have sought to increase their influence in and control over health care (Larkin, 1988). Concurrently, allied health professionals have sought a greater say in what kinds of health care should be available.

Status differences and delegating

Traditionally, the different hierarchies within a health care organization were more concerned with communication among themselves, than with other hierarchies. Medical, nursing, and allied professions all had their own hierarchy, though the latest reorganization of the National Health Service (NHS) in the UK, and the Hosptial Authority in Hong Kong for example has to an extent reduced this somewhat, with organization shifting to units and away from professions. Despite this, doctors still direct doctors (and sometimes other groups), nurses direct nurses, and so on.

Between professions, the relationship between doctors and nurses has traditionally been one of doctors delegating specified tasks to nurses and directing nurses in their activities, while nurses have been responsible for carrying out these instructions. This is the ward model. In other work environments, such as operating theatres, nurses work in a much more integrated fashion with the surgeons. This style of work is much more collaborative than ward work. These two contexts illustrate different types of interaction. There are clearly many other different styles of interaction, some of which are more role-specific than others. In an accident and emergency department or coronary care unit for example, nurses may act more independently in carrying out tasks.

Increasingly, many medical doctors are recognizing that they are one profession among many in delivering health care. Yet the issue of patient responsibility still affects the relationship between medical and other professional groups. This is seen most clearly in multidisciplinary team care. When a multidisciplinary team is established, there is an assumption that the doctor is the leader. This is despite the fact that the doctor is so short of time and may not be the best person, being overqualified, so to speak, for the job. This is true in areas such as rehabilitative care, chronic disease management teams, community care, and many other areas.

It is hardly surprising that, with these pressures, some senior members of the medical profession feel under threat. They are seen as legally responsible, so they are trapped into being 'in charge' although this can cause major difficulties. Compare a nursing unit manager with many years of experience in intensive care and a newly appointed house officer in terms of practical experience about intensive care. The doctor has the responsibility, but probably less knowledge. The nursing officer, usually tactfully, guides the doctor into the correct course of action and tries to prevent the doctor from making mistakes. The wise house officer recognizes the expertise of other professionals and finds time to communicate with them.

Control and care

Szasz and Hollander (1965) classified the nature of relationships between doctors and patients into three broad styles: active/passive, guidance/ co-operation, and mutual participation. The styles of work relationships outlined above can also be classified according to the Szasz and Hollander model. Styles of communication between different professionals are influenced by the attitudes and relationships that prevail among these different professionals. Freeling (1986) quoted Dame Catherine Hall, former President of the United Kingdom Central Council for Nursing (UKCC) of nursing professions as believing 'There is a general feeling in the nursing profession that the majority of doctors still retain a stereotyped image of the nurse as one who is to do their bidding . . . Where the stereotyped image of nursing is still held problems in communication are inevitable.' (Freeling, 1986). A prime example of this kind of attitude, though in relation this time to social workers, is given by Kessel (1986). '(The doctor) . . . will not tolerate interference from others who are not team members', and 'Doctors tend to assume that, if there is a team of which they are a member, they will be in charge . . . It must remain so in the field of medicine, and if other health professionals do not like it they must lump it.' (Kessel, 1986). It is unfortunate that these attitudes appear in a book aimed at improving communication between doctors and others in the caring professions.

The mutually participative approach to team work will be by far the most successful if enacted in an agreed style.

Underlying these poor communications are attitudes about relationships with other professionals. Though doctors are exemplified as poor communicators, they are not the only health care professionals with problems of communications. Within professions also, different specialities can lead to similar perceived differences in status (e.g. between speciality-trained nurses and non-speciality-trained nurses on a ward), between different types of therapists (e.g. physiotherapists versus occupational therapists), or between similar professional groups (e.g. psychiatrists, psychologists, psychiatric social workers and nurse therapists) and so on.

Hazards of poor communication between staff

Clinical

The most important hazard of poor communications between health professionals is the risk to the patient. Communication breakdown puts the patient at risk. Because of the constraints on face-to-face communication outlined above, health workers must rely on the clinical record as the main source of information about current status and planned care of a patient. Yet anyone who has tried to read a set of case notes immediately faces the problems inherent in the traditional written case notes. The whole area of written records in health care is currently in a mess. One of the greatest priorities needed in health care is to organize an efficient and comprehensive form of recorded information about patients that improves communication.

It is almost impossible to wade through three-volume sets of case notes of patients who have been deeply enmeshed in the health care system for years, and to understand innumerable different specialists with their own shorthand for tests and diagnoses. There are plenty of requests and often too much information, and for some case notes there is probably no one person capable of deciphering everything they contain. The danger of such notes is that they contain too much memoranda, legal protection and other information that does not communicate meaningfully to others.

Information technology promises changes to the way records are kept. It is pointless to simply reproduce the chaotic system of written records in electronic form. There is a flurry of research and anxiety about how best to present clinical information in electronic form. Distributed networking looks promising. This involves, for example, a number of computer nodes, with terminals in the ward, laboratory, out-patient clinic, all of which have their own record, but which could be accessed from each of the other sites. Thus, the ward could get information from the laboratory as soon as available, together with previous test results, in different representations (numerical, graphical). The laboratory record would not contain the same information as the ward record, which could include diagnostic, treatment and outcome information. Different levels of security could be provided so that confidential patient information was only available to persons involved in patient care. This applies as much to nursing as to medical information (Swenson-Feldman and Brugge-Wiger, 1985).

For most of us, this paperless case record will be several years away, though it will be here sooner rather than later. In the meantime, improving written case records should be a priority.

Litigation

The increasing frequency of litigation over what is seen as health care malpractice or negligence is closely associated with poor communications. Doctors and nurses who do not communicate with their patients (and with each other) are more likely to be involved in litigation than those who do communicate. Twenty-seven percent of medicolegal cases in one region of the UK were found to be associated with problems in communication (Hawkins and Paterson, 1987). The same seems to apply in the USA (Larkin, 1988).

Staff litigation and union problems are also more likely in organizations with poor communications. The nature of this poor communication is likely to be associated with the non-availability of professional managers, the labelling of staff members as problematic, low morale, and mushroom management (being kept in the dark and having muck dropped on you).

Professional stagnation

On a more personal level, poor professional development, low staff morale and difficulties in motivating staff have already been mentioned as consequences. Stagnation of staff was commonly seen in large psychiatric hospitals where it was called institutionalization. Institutionalization is a reason to close down the large asylums (though economics plays a role). Many staff who had worked for years in such places were themselves as institutionalized as the patients. There are hazards among certain types of chronic care. The level of care provided is less than optimal; staff may feel there is little they can do other than toileting, bed making and drug distributing. Where geographic isolation also occurs, this can compound the sense of psychological and professional isolation.

When morale is low, people 'get sick' of working, leading to greater absenteeism. This increases demand on other staff, compounding lack of staff development. Low morale also has a negative effect on patient care (Revans, 1964). Staff who are low in morale are more difficult to work with. Attitudes or behaviour of other staff is the most frequent source of complaint heard from nurses (McIntee and Firth, 1984).

Higher operating costs and inefficiencies

The inefficiencies arising from poor communication are significant. From an administrative perspective, absenteeism and staff turnover are costly. So is union strife and personal litigation. Poor communication is costly in other ways, such as inappropriate requests of tests or treatments. The use of investigations has been increasing almost exponentially over the past decade. There has long been a worrying body of evidence suggesting that most of these investigations are unnecessary and that they do not lead to changes in patient health (Palmer, 1985).

This increase in investigations is very costly in resource terms. This in part reflects lack of communication between doctors and the staff who carry out the investigation. Laboratory staff, for example, are often in a better position to advise a doctor (especially a house officer) on the value of certain tests, yet they are seldom consulted. Similarly, doctors (or nurses or even ward clerks) who complete request forms frequently fail to provide important information on the request form that is needed by the laboratory. Many doctors fail to realize that laboratory staff need certain clinical information on request forms (e.g. menstrual history on curettage specimens sent for analysis) (Whimster, 1986).

A test result on a form may take three to five days, sometimes over a week from being requested to reaching the requesting doctor. Delays are often practical (postal problems; case notes moved somewhere else; wrong media or anticoagulant used for the test required). The lab may then get a second or third request (from casualty, the ward and outpatients). Case notes being such a mess, it can sometimes take a long time to locate a previous test result. Whereas health service reforms try to contain costs, they fail to address these inefficiencies arising from communication issues.

These are powerful reasons to improve communications not only between patients and health workers, but also between health workers themselves. Let us now explore some of the main problems in intra-professional communications.

▆ Barriers to professional communications

Within the same profession

Communications within the same profession can be considered as three distinct areas: clinical, educational and administrative. Clinical communications involve communications with members of the same profession, who may be on different shifts, or are members of a different team or speciality. Two areas are explored: written letters of referral and report, and changes in shift or responsibility for patients. Educational communications occur in clinical training of members in the same profession. Examples are individual training in specific skills, and presentation of research findings to colleagues. Administrative communications are those communications involving managerial/administrative activities. Educational and administrative/managerial communications are outside the scope of this book and are not considered further.

What are the main reasons why members of the same profession might not communicate well with one another? The list of reasons can include:

1. lack of availability
2. evaluation instead of feedback
3. lack of consultation/control
4. exclusion from decisions
5. lack of agreed guidelines
6. lack of regular affirmative feedback
7. competitiveness or rivalry
8. inadequate records

Some of these factors are self-explanatory. Staff who are not available are difficult to communicate with. There has been little research into availability of health workers as a barrier to communication. Following a study of the ease of contacting duty doctors responsible for emergency admissions, Bakhai et al (1990) concluded that the availability and response time of these doctors 'seemed fairly easy' when switchboards were used. However, during daytime, a doctor who is responsible for patients in a number of wards, and who is also working in an outpatient clinic may be only accessible by phone, and then only some of the time. For surgeons who are in operating theatres, a colleague may cover for them, though this does not always happen in practice.

The importance of feedback instead of evaluation has already been discussed. Health workers who are continually evaluative in their collegial communications makes others feel uncomfortable. Staff then avoid communicating with such individuals. Middle managers who are selectively evaluative in their collegial communications generate strong feelings of resentment among some staff and strong loyalties among others. From a managerial perspective, the resulting split in ward cohesiveness is undesirable and should be identified and addressed by training in managerial communications. Feedback can serve the same purpose as evaluation, but is less hierarchical and more affirmative.

Feeling a part of the organization is important for all staff. Feeling in control is as important for health workers at all levels, as it is for patients. It is important to feel able to influence things to bring about change if necessary. Where clinical practice approaches are laid down by one or two people, the majority who have to implement the practice may find problems and difficulties which were not anticipated. Under good working conditions, an individual can go back to the planners and provide feedback on the problem. The approach can then be adjusted to take this problem into account. If this procedure seems familiar, it should. It is the basic model for the improvement of any system and manifests itself in many forms — in clinical intervention research, in the nursing process, and in management development strategies.

However, in many health establishments, the hierarchical nature of the management structure means that the flow of information is predominantly downwards, or that little notice is given to feedback from the clinical level. Major problems can exist in manager visibility, feedback and staff recognition and participation in decision making (Townsend, 1991). This results in individuals feeling their input is undervalued, except as a pair of hands, and thus their commitment to excellence can become impaired.

The lack of agreed guidelines on communication policy can also lead to difficulties. Where hierarchical management systems exist, it is assumed that communications are made through line management, that is, to and from an immediate superior and junior. For cross-communications about patient care, the ward round, ward meeting ('handover') and case conference are the formal means of exchanging information between colleagues. However, there may be a lack of agreed guidelines for informal communications, during night-shifts or at other times outside such meetings.

Finally, competitiveness, rivalry or interpersonal disputes are common barriers to communications. These can be some of the most difficult problems to address, especially if they occur among more senior personnel. Patients deteriorate drastically while particular doctors refuse to seek an opinion from a specialist with whom they have been in contention with. Rivalries can last for decades. For some reason, academics seem most vulnerable to these kinds of interpersonal rivalries, though by no means exclusively.

Finally, poor case records also impair communications between members of the same profession. These problems have already been raised and will not be repeated. Suffice it to say that the case record is, first and foremost, a communications resource, not simply a note book or legal cover for a particular practitioner.

Between different professions

Most, if not all, of the problems outlined in the last section also apply to communications between different professional groups. In addition, the question of written communications will be dealt with here, though much of what is important in this area also applies to communications between members of the same profession (especially in the case of medical staff).

There are two written means of communication which are important but that have not yet been discussed. These are the referral letter and the subsequent report to the referring agency. One problem with cross-disciplinary communications that doesn't arise (at least as frequently) among members of the same profession is the jargon language barrier. Recall that part of becoming a health worker involves acquiring the language of the particular profession. Jargon is most pronounced in medicine, but also is found among nurses, psychologists and other allied health professionals. In face-to-face communication clarification can be made. Other professionals may not ask for clarification of jargon for fear of being thought ignorant. In written communication, this can be more difficult and time consuming. A second, and more important problem is lack of clarity in written communications.

Communications between mental health professionals and others are often problematic. Leonard, Babbs and Creed (1990) reported that 20% of 200 referral letters to psychiatrists did not express the precise reason why psychiatric opinion was sought and many psychiatrists' replies did not describe adequately the follow-up arrangements and prognosis. In general, psychiatrists found the referral letters short and lacking in information. On the other hand, half of the referring doctors expressed preferences for replies that were one-page long letters and contained key items of information with clear psychiatric diagnosis and opinion, and clear treatment/follow-up arrangements. The findings in this study must be assumed to apply to other areas.

Facilitating professional communications

Models of communication

The traditional theory of communication is derived from the SMCR (Sender, Message, Code, Receiver) theory (Shannon and Weaver, 1949). This has purposefully not been discussed because it over-simplifies human face-to-face communication. Despite this, it has provided the basis for many books on communication between people. People, it should come as no surprise, are more complex than radios (and computers). But they are also self-aware. It is this point that makes the SMCR theory mostly irrelevant for present purposes.

A comprehensive theory of communication needs to take in to account not simply a mechanical model like SMCR, but must consider the psychological realities of the communicators, the nature of the communication, and the contexts. The problem of attitude in professional communications has been raised. It is also clear that people who disagree tend to work less well together. When coerced into following someone else's idea, people seldom do their best work (Hamilton, 1987). Communication can both help to achieve mutual understanding and be facilitated by such understanding.

A more realistic model is the convergence model of communication (Kincaid, 1986). Briefly, this theory suggests communications can enhance (or degrade) organizational function through mutual understanding in the process of deliberate change. Central to this model is the belief that communication involves common perceptions, interpretations and beliefs. This leads to effective joint action towards shared goals. We assume the need for shared respect and mutually positive attitudes towards each person in the communication exchange.

General strategies for improving communications

From an organizational perspective, improving communications within a professional group or team is best achieved once the current communication patterns are known. The approach used to gather this information is the same as that used to evaluate any activity. First, an assessment is made, then on the basis of this assessment a plan of action is developed and implemented. A subsequent assessment is then carried out to evaluate whether the desired outcome has been achieved. This procedure can go through any number of iterations, until the outcome is to everybody's satisfaction.

The manager who decides that the communications in a given unit are in need of improvement can approach the problem by carrying out a 'communications audit'. This is the same as a financial audit, but it traces the flow of communication around an organization, instead of money. When whole organizations are in need of such an audit, specialists are best employed for the purpose (Hamilton, 1987). For most cases, a more modest approach than that advocated by Hamilton is called for.

Irrespective of the level and scope of the interventions chosen, evaluation both before and after is necessary to assess the impact of any changes.

Key Points
Before implementing any changes, assess the current situation. Then, on the basis of the data obtained from this assessment, plan and implement changes. Finally, follow up with a repeat of the assessment to check that the goals have been achieved.

Improving communications within the same profession

Many of the principles already discussed in previous chapters apply just as much to communication between colleagues as between health worker and patient. Relevant chapters to review are those on interviewing, especially sections on how to ask questions, listening, empathy, dealing with emotions, and giving information. These skills constitute an important part of communications between people generally.

There are several things that unit managers can do to facilitate communications between their staff. These include the following:

1. policy statement
2. regular meetings
3. availability of senior staff for consultation
4. being sensitive to staff needs for support and advice
5. providing orientation for new staff
6. consulting staff regularly
7. delegating
8. participating as a person
9. newsletter
10. adopting optimal work methods

Policy statement.   A policy statement is not really a statement as such. Instead, it is a general information resource for all people on the unit. What is given should be agreed on and written, then posted on the unit notice board. This board, in effect, serves as the policy statement. It should specify key information about communication on the unit. This will include an organizational chart of the unit. This could give a clearly posted list of all staff working on the unit with a sliding cover specifying whether currently on or off duty. This is useful to inform visitors to the ward as well as other staff as to who is working.

Also included in the policy statement would be the name of the staff member in charge of any particular team or shift, names of staff responsible for particular roles, the name of the next manager on duty up the management line and other important information of this nature. This is also a clear statement of certain responsibilities.

Finally, a policy statement should include some information about times of meetings and statements aimed to encourage unit personnel to submit written suggestions or comments for meetings if they are unable to attend. A suggestion box could also be provided. The policy statement can go a long way to meeting many of the facilitative points in the list above.

Regular meetings.   Regular meetings are an important part of the unit communication process. These can be of two types, in addition to the ward handover or case-conference meeting. These are specific meetings to discuss unit policy, development and progress, and specific meetings held to develop communications, provide support or build team spirit.

Policy meetings might be held monthly or quarterly and unit managers might invite their manager to attend in order that staff can access this next level of management directly. In these meetings, staff are encouraged to provide input aimed at developing the unit performance. This input may take the form of a discussion of procedures for certain activities undertaken by the unit; it may involve an academic presentation by a member of the unit or by someone from outside talking about a different approach. The meeting would provide a venue for staff to discuss and agree on policies and responsibilities, and to clarify uncertainties. Thus it would serve as both policy and staff development venue. It might be held at lunch time as a kind of brown-bag meeting.

Support meetings, in contrast, are convened specifically to encourage a strengthening of the unit socially and emotionally. Certain infrequent occurrences, such as disasters, can place excessive demand on staff. Following this type of event, it may be helpful to run a group for a short period of time to help staff deal with the powerful feelings that major trauma can evoke. It is important to provide good support during such times and not just afterwards. This area is discussed more fully below.

Delegation, participation and information.   Three further suggestions for improving communication are delegation of responsibilities, participation in unit activity, and providing full access to information.

Delegation of responsibility is an important act. It not only infers trust and acknowledgement of a person's ability, but also serves to encourage communication through regular consultation exchanges with the delegate, and the delegate with others. Once work has been delegated, let the delegate get on with it. Don't interfere unless requested to. Participation in unit activity involves the senior members of the unit carrying out activities alongside the most junior. Not only do the junior members learn from such experiences, but they make possible a more ready exchange of communication that might otherwise not occur. Finally, the provision of information to staff, with the opportunity for discussion is of key importance. It increases predictability, and gives an opportunity for others to gather information or feedback ideas on the information. This kind of information giving has been shown to have the most beneficial effect on unit climates (James, Milne and Firth, 1990). This in turn improves staff retention (Hart and Moore, 1989).

As with patient communication, *how* something is said can be more important than *what* is said. As staff in a health care facility, there is no one but other staff to turn to for support. Feeling valued professionally and personally is important for good morale and a happy working environment. It also facilitates high standards of work.

Adoption of optimal working strategies.   Adoption of optimal work strategies also facilitates communication. Work strategies that focus on task achievement are often less satisfying to staff than those which hand over responsibility for setting priorities for care. Task-oriented work in health care is the equivalent of assembly line work. Individuals specialize in carrying out tasks, sometimes with great regularity, but have little input otherwise to the planning and evaluation of patient care.

The traditional style of nursing exemplifies this. The principal tasks were seen as taking temperatures and blood pressures, 'toileting', giving out drugs, etc. The work day consisted of a sequence of tasks to be worked through in a particular order. Not only is such an approach fundamentally unsatisfying to the nurse carrying out the task, it can be stressful and leaves little room for important aspects of nursing care, such as interacting with the patient. Given that many of the tasks that nurses carry out — often to doctors' orders — may offer limited benefit to the patient, and have little bearing on the subsequent management of the patient, they can be deemed largely unnecessary (Burroughs and Hoffbrand, 1990).

However, it can be particularly difficult to implement a change of practice towards a more efficient working strategy, such as primary nursing and reflective practice. The new approach may generate problems of it own (Weeks, Barrett and Snead, 1985), and it is not simply sufficient to announce a change and then implement it. Often a structured training programme needs to be introduced to effect and retain changes, particularly in those staff resistant to new methods (Seto, Ching, Fung and Fielding, 1989). However, once such changes are implemented, they can lead to improved communication and collaboration on the unit (McMahon, 1990).

Other approaches include having a unit newsletter to inform staff of interesting research and practice developments, availability of training opportunities, refresher courses, etc.

Facilitating communications between different health professions.   Communications between different health care professions are generally more problematic than those between members of the same profession. Often, the perspective of a problem differs due to the differing backgrounds of the two workers. This may present problems when it comes to defining the nature of a problem to be solved. A social worker may perceive a problem in social terms while a doctor may perceive the same problem in biological terms. A second set of problems that have already been outlined in the introduction to this chapter arise from status differences and role conflicts.

These reflect differences in attitude towards one another and the associated responsibilities. Thus, a doctor may be critical of nurses who exceed their professional role by making their own diagnosis.

Adopting collaborative practice.   Differences in practice styles may then lead to problems. The adoption of collaborative practice as an alternative style of providing hospital-based care is promising. Bradford (1989) has identified developments necessary in both medical and nursing professions for the successful implementation of collaborative care. These are for nurses:

- primary nursing
- reflective nursing
- integrated charting (nurses and doctors use one problem-oriented medical record)
- expanded nurses decision making
- joint patient care review
- collaborative communications monitored through committee
- developing assertiveness
- improving their knowledge of the care of their patients
- developing effective communication patterns with physicians

For the medical staff, a change to more collaborative working means:

- gaining greater understanding of professional nursing practice
- avoiding aggressive behaviour towards nurses
- developing professional security and maturity based on collaboration not domination
- supporting the adoption of integrated charting

Many of these practices are already present in fragmentary ways, with the exception of the more formal recognition and establishment by committee of the monitoring process. Once the decision is made jointly between management of both medical and nursing groups, consultation with the unit staff should follow and a pilot project could be run to identify problems. It should be agreed beforehand to implement this style of practice. The pilot project serves to identify obstacles to its implementation which are then tackled and solved. The problems encountered in pilot projects should not be used as excuses to abandon the implementation of such practice. Sabotage is easy otherwise. It may be necessary to set up a small (three-person) group to deal with inter-discipline problems, but once implemented, benefits to staff communication (and patient care) are substantial (Bradford, 1989).

Using job descrptions to develop new practice styles is very important, particularly in specifying role responsibilities in terms of non-clinical care roles, for example, in research nurses or for roles involving collaboration management.

Improving record keeping. On a communications level, the adoption of an integrated problem-oriented medical record is most important. This would contain input from all the different professions involved in patient care. To keep in touch with a patient's care, each professional would have to read the input of other professionals.

It is envisaged that this record would, in the first instance, be a written record. Ultimately, however, the record would be computerized into some form of integrated information system. The nature of the medical record is the subject of much investigation and development. It needs to be concise first and foremost without sacrificing accuracy, clarity or flexibility. The nature of this record must be highly structured in both written and electronic forms to facilitate both the recording and extraction of information. This structure is an inherent part of a good record, providing a prompt for certain procedures as well as providing specific areas for recording clinical details (McGhee, 1990).

This is not the place to go into the details of patient record systems but some potential advantages of a centralized and structured information system (besides improving practitioner communications) include:

- evaluation of the process of care and outcome
- important information in the record less likely to be overlooked
- prompts for screening, tests, etc. (continuity of care) built in
- laboratory report immediately accessible
- arrangement of outpatient, ambulance, etc. bookings facilitated
- bed availability immediately accessible
- quality control and costing benefits
- patient billing facilitated
- production of reports and data in different forms (e.g. graphical)

Assertiveness. Assertiveness is not aggression. Assertiveness is the process of asserting: to defend one's rights or opinions. To be assertive one has to feel positively about oneself and one's rights. Low self-esteem is sometimes linked to the socialization of women which can carry over to the work place. The system of nursing education may also encourage low self-esteem (Bradford, 1989). The role dominance hierarchy of male doctors and female nurses may make assertiveness even more difficult.

The area of assertiveness training is extensive and constitutes a range of theory too substantial to detail here. Interested readers should consult the many texts available on this subject.

Feedback and empathy.   An important key in assertiveness is to provide feedback to others and to demonstrate empathy with their position or view, whilst maintaining your own. The advantage of feedback over evaluation has been discussed in the introduction to this chapter. When used in an empathic manner feedback is a powerful way of providing information to others while indicating a sensitivity to their circumstances. Consider the following example:

Nurse 1:   I'll get those test forms done now

Dr: Thanks, I'll see you at the unit meeting on Friday . . .

Nurse 2:   Excuse me Dr Smith, I can see you're busy but I think it is important that we talk about Mrs Jones.

Dr: Can you do half hourly obs? I think we'd better keep a close eye on her.

Nurse: Mrs Jones' has asked to speak to you. I don't think she will be conscious much longer. It's important you talk with her.

Dr: Look, I've got a clinic and I'm already ten minutes late. Could you find out what she wants and I'll try and call in later tonight?

Nurse: I think she would appreciate telling you herself.

Dr: Once she starts I'll be there for ages.

Nurse: If you talk with her briefly now and tell her you can spend more time this evening maybe that will satisfy her for now. I'll talk with her in the meantime.

Dr: (Sigh) Ok. I'll do that.

Nurse: Are half-hourly observations really necessary for Mrs Jones? I have two other poorly patients to care for and my time with her could be better spent than doing temps and BPs.

Dr: I suppose hourly would do if you keep an eye on her.

Nurse: That makes my job easier. It'll be better for her too. I'll page you if there are any changes. One more thing. After your talk with Mrs Jones tonight, can we sit down for ten minutes and plan her care?

Dr: OK. I'll be here about six, but if I don't go now it'll be midnight before I finish.

In this exchange, the nurse demonstrated both empathic statements ('I can see you're very busy') and feedback ('I think she would appreciate telling you herself'; 'That makes my job easier'). There is also appropriate assertiveness ('I think she would appreciate telling you herself') in these statements: when the doctor tried to avoid responsibilities, the nurse pressed the importance of the doctor seeing the patient, albeit briefly.

Arranging availability. The above example also illustrated availability to communicate. Being available is a necessity for communication. Scheduled meeting times are one way of improving availability for communications purposes. However, in the management of seriously ill patients, it may be necessary for the doctor and nurse who are primarily involved in the patient's care to meet on a daily basis, perhaps only for five minutes or so at a time, but frequently. Again, the use of a central problem-oriented medical record can facilitate this substantially.

Written communications. Written communications in the form of letters of referral and reports are facilitated by computerized problem-oriented medical records. It is a simple matter to print out a brief set of relevant data selected from the record to accompany the written letter or referral or report, or better still, to arrange access to the record by the party to whom the patient has been referred. Research on letters of referral suggests that the following features are preferred:
- make letters succinct (one page is optimal)
- organize material into meaningful categories
- avoid specialist jargon, neologisms, initials, e.g. BMDP
- make available the (summarized) record subsequently
- provide relevant medical and other information, especially diagnosis
- clearly specify the reason for referral

Similarly, for reports, a printout from a problem-oriented medical record can provide a supplement of laboratory and other investigations. The report letter itself should have the following features:
- brief, clear and precise — about one page in length and with main points highlighted
- without specialist jargon, initials, etc.
- with recommendations clearly stated

Giving information to non-professionals

The principles that apply to giving information to non-professionals are the same as those for other health professionals. Namely, first and foremost, organize your information into meaningful units. Then use repetition and emphasis to ensure the main points are recalled. Use explicit categorization (see Chapter 9), together with other techniques for increasing recall. A review of the points in Chapters 9 and 10 is recommended.

Communications with the media

Occasionally, it may be necessary to meet with the press or other media representative, such as television, who are interested in the work of the unit or particular patients undergoing new treatment.

There are pitfalls associated with media communications. Editors are employed by publishers to sell their publication. It is not unusual for a complex issue to be explained in a clear and careful manner to a reporter, only to have an editor or sub-editor re-write the copy out of all recognition. This is usually done to make a 'story' more attractive to other publications (who may then buy it) and to the reader. For obvious reasons, it is more difficult to re-write a taped interview. However, taped interviews can be cut in creative ways to highlight the dramatic or controversial elements and remove or relegate any reservations or qualifying statements cautiously added.

Insist that you be allowed to read and amend the final copy before it is submitted to print. The widespread availability of fax machines makes this quite feasible. Even where there is no fax, telephones will do as a last resort. No agency has reason to refuse such a request. If this is refused, consider withdrawing permission for the interview to be used. Chances are, it will not be recognizable. But bear in mind, a reported or editor is under no compulsion to remove any copy, despite objections from yourself. It is less easy to review a tape recorded interview prior to broadcasting, especially if it is 'hot' news, as this may be aired upon receipt by the media. Reviewing may be possible if the material forms part of a documentary or similar programme. These dire warnings aside, how does one deal with the scrupulous media reporter or press conference to minimize the misunderstanding or misquotation? There are several basic approaches already outlined that can be adapted to the press conference format.

First, it is worth taking the time and effort to produce a press release, which in your own, or agreed words, should clearly specify the following:
- A brief introduction orienting the lay reader to the nature of the topic. This may include some simple statistics in understandable form, such as the incidence of a particular condition.
- The main points you wish to get across in an itemized fashion, clearly separated from one another.
- Any limitations or conditions associated with the information already given, including exclusions and contradictions for a proposed new treatment, for example.

The press release should be given out at the beginning of the press conference. Questions can then be taken to clarify the material present in the handout where necessary. Reporters often try to lead a person to expand on a cautious statement, for example. Try to avoid being lead to speculate beyond the points you have already specified. Refer the questioner to the press release. Don't be afraid to admit when you do not know the limitations or outcome. Though you may want to express your hopes or expectations, specify that these are not 'facts'.

In an individual interview (one-to-one) situation, which will be much more likely for most health workers, it is worth going over with the reporter the area of interest before exploring more specific questions.

Avoid using jargon. This is usually misunderstood by non-specialist journalists and is a major source of confusion. Ask the journalist to read back any technical explanations and check for clarity and accuracy.

Above all, try to be well prepared for the interview. It can be very embarrassing to be asked a simple question that you should be able to answer and not have the information available. Try to remain relaxed and avoid catastrophic thinking ('This will be awful!', 'I'll never cope!', 'What will I say if they ask me xyz?'). This will only make you more anxious. Instead, try to rehearse the interview with a friend or colleague beforehand. The friend can play the part of the reporter and you can practise answering the questions in a range of different ways until you feel more comfortable. You friend can also provide useful feedback on your responses to their questions.

Reducing stress and providing support through communications

Providing for the emotional well-being of staff requires recognition of the situations and circumstances that stress may become a problem for health workers. Recognizing stressful units and events is an important managerial skill. But individual health workers are more important for giving support in an informal, day-to-day fashion than specified groups or systems.

Work-related stress often arises from poor communications. The adoption of stereotyped attitudes about people or other professionals (e.g. All doctors are arrogant! All nurses are dumb!), and misunderstandings about the working practices of others confound this. It is not unusual to hear health workers complain about the administration not doing their job properly, or taking too much time to get something done. By contrast, the process of dealing with external businesses and suppliers, and the often unpredictable fluctuations in markets are seldom understood by health workers in a clinic.

Among the most difficult types of situation for staff to deal with are those where there is unpredictability or where control is otherwise reduced. Even low level background stress can be debilitating, interfering with people's ability to work efficiently, straining relationships, and causing higher levels of sickness, absenteeism and staff turnover.

Talking with people informally, usually while carrying out work activities, is the most common way that staff perceive support from colleagues (McIntee and Firth, 1984). By making adjustments to care practices so that workers are not left to work on their own can result in improved performance, communications and staff satisfaction (Weeks, Barrett and Snead, 1985).

McIntee and Firth (1984) compared British and American nursing staff, both qualified and unqualified and asked the questions 'Who has been most supportive?' and 'How have they been most supportive?' Communication skill was consistently reported as the most important reason for people being supportive. Specifically, skills including the following were most important:

- giving information or explanation
- giving suggestions or advice
- listening, understanding, getting me to talk
- showing an interest in me or my work

Behaviour and attitudes of other staff were constantly reported as the most stressful aspects of the work in this study. The authors commented on the striking degree of consistency in responses from both junior and senior staff.

It seems, therefore, that good support can be provided without the use of organized support programmes. Expression of support can be encouraged by adopting work practices that put people together to work in teams or groups, preventing isolation. By exploring attitudes to other professional groups, and by the use of some of the communications strategies outlined earlier in this chapter.

Group support programmes

Support meetings have been argued to be especially important on units where there is a high level of emotional demand, such as paediatric oncology units. However, few studies have looked at this and there is some uncertainty as to whether the benefits of organizing such groups are worth the effort involved (Tyson et al, 1984). Support can also be effectively provided for staff in an informal fashion, during normal activities, among which communication skills are major contributors (McIntee and Firth, 1984).

For some types of work, such as AIDS units, support groups may provide a means of helping colleagues cope with some of the difficulties in the work. AIDS can raise major psychosocial issues among staff, especially those working with AIDS patients for the first time (Pasacreta and Jacobsen, 1989). In such cases, some kind of support system is probably needed.

Providing support should involve the following skills:

- being available
- attending and listening, showing interest
- encouraging the expression of concerns
- encouraging confidence in ideas of others
- giving feedback instead of evaluation
- providing information
- giving advice or suggestions when asked for
- respecting confidentiality of discussion

Whether this is done privately between two people or in a group setting makes no difference. It seems that these are the skills most likely to be perceived as supportive by other staff (McIntee and Firth, 1984).

Summary

- Staff communications can be task-oriented or performance/self oriented.
- Feedback is non-evaluative information on some aspect of performance/self.
- Uncertainty about role expectations and standards can lead to confusion about task or personal performance.
- Poor staff communications affect stress levels and morale of staff, resulting in high absenteeism and high staff turnover.
- Reasons for poor inter-professional communications include:
  - role conflict
  - perceived threats to professional integrity
  - status differences and task delegation conflicts
  - reactionary attitudes
  - inadequate case note formats

- Poor communications result in
  - increased risk of patient litigation
  - impaired staff development
  - higher staff turnover and absenteeism
  - increased costs
- Implementing communications change involves
  - assessing the current situation
  - planning and implementing changes based on the assessment
  - following up with a repeat of the assessment to check that the goals have been achieved
- Collaborative practice and problem-oriented records facilitate communication between different professions.
- Written material should be concise, brief and the main points underlined.
- Use of assertiveness, feedback and empathic statements retains access to other staff and improves effectiveness.
- Give information according to the principles stated in chapter 9.
- Provide press releases for press conferences and be prepared for interviews with reporters.
- Avoid technical terms and give simple statistics with meaning for benefit of non-technical media.
- Minimize staff stress by
  - warm, open communications
  - provide advice to less experience colleagues
  - show an interest in the person and their work
- Providing support involves:
  - availability
  - attending and listening, showing interest
  - encouraging the expression of concerns
  - encouraging confidence in ideas of others
  - giving feedback instead of evaluation
  - providing information
  - giving advice or suggestions when asked for
  - respecting confidentiality of discussion

Exercises

Some of these exercises are for use among small groups as they focus on group interaction.

As with previous exercises, participation will ensure the maximum benefit.

1. Work in groups of three. Your task is to identify an area of professional communications in your place of work which you think could be either a source of problems or which has caused misunderstandings in the past. Using your knowledge of communications try to discover why these problems occur and ways that these problems can be overcome (by use of written schedules, meetings, planning, re-organization of work etc.). Spend 15 minutes thinking about your own problem and trying to come up with solutions. After 15 minutes, each take turns in sharing your solutions with the other two group members. Give feedback on the suggestions of the other two group members in turn. Spend up to10 minutes each discussing your proposals. When you have completed the exercise, take another 5 minutes to incorporate ideas into your solution. Then, two groups team up to form a group of six and choose one area from each of the two groups to discuss again. Take up to 15 minutes.

2. Record keeping. Working alone, consider what the most common problems in managing written information on patients are in your work. Write down what these are. Discuss these problems in your group. Try to identify ways they can be overcome or reduced. How many of you identified the same kinds of problems?

3   Consider your approach to discussing with a colleague/other professional/manager a grievance you have. Can you identify any tendencies you have which may impair your ability to get your point across to the other person in a constructive way? What could you do to smooth the discussion. Spend 5 minutes on this.

4. Role play with a colleague the following: You feel you have been unfairly treated regarding your work schedule and want to discuss this with your manager. Be yourself. Your task is to try to get your manager to change your schedule. The manager's task is to resist such a change because this will cause quite a lot of work. Spend 10 minutes on this.

Discussion

1. What are the disadvantages of introducing integrated record keeping in your unit/centre/hospital? How many of these disadvantages are practical and how many attitudinal?

2. What would be the advantages and disadvantages of setting up support groups in your unit/centre/hospital?

3. Should patients be allowed to have free access to the data kept on them during hospitalization (including medical and nursing records)? If not, why not?

14

Concluding Remarks

As you read this book, you may have gathered the impression that it was written with a bias towards change. This was the intention. A system that has in many ways failed to provide adequately for its consumers on one level while becoming over reliant on the technological level warrants change. The adoption of communications as a priority form of care can be justified from many different points of view. Once adopted, however, it becomes increasingly difficult to maintain old ways of working. It brings about a revolution ultimately leading to more and more person-oriented health care, away from rigid and secretive styles that dominate and threaten while claiming to care. As consumers become more knowledgeable, they expect higher levels of service, and where these are not forthcoming, dissatisfied people resort to other means, such as litigation, to achieve their goals.

In communicating more extensively and more sensitively, greater priority is given to psychological, social and emotional aspects of ill health and care. As a consequence, health care systems become more humane and people-oriented. It requires a shift in priorities to achieve this, just as it requires a shift in attitudes to develop communications competence, to recognize that time spent talking with a patient is *not* time wasted.

Of course, one problem is that despite the best efforts of health workers and educationalists, people generally give little thought to their health until they become sick. At such times, many go to the doctor for a quick fix, having adopted simple, mechanistic views of health and illness. These attitudes are not going to change overnight, but honest open communication will help to emphasize greater awareness of self care.

These changes in the attitudes of health professionals and patients must be accompanied by other changes towards viewing patients as autonomous individuals ultimately responsible for their own health. This in turn indicates that more emphasis on encouraging participation in decision making and care is needed. So, we move away from paternalistic medicine and maternalistic nursing care to a situation where patients are encouraged to become responsible experts in their own health, with expert guidance. When this happens, people may then begin to change their practices and become more health conscious.

Communication acts to subvert the distance between patient and practitioner. It is unashamedly a tool for political change, as every government knows; whoever controls communication, controls the state. On a more mundane level, it is a tool for changing our working environment, to make us less isolated by professionalism and more accessible to patients and each other. It brings with it as a natural extension, recognition of a more general level of human interaction, what has been called whole-person care, and a change in practice from disease control to true health care.

Thus, to summarize the main points that I hope the reader will take away from reading this book:

1. Adopting communications care as a priority in health care delivery is likely to significantly improve patient satisfaction, adherence to treatment, treatment effectiveness and consequently health outcomes (assuming the treatments are not themselves detrimental in the first place).

2. By adopting ADA models of information giving, under or over disclosure of information can easily be avoided, thereby optimizing information exchange. This can facilitate diagnosis and treatment and further enhance mutual satisfaction with care.

3. Appropriate communications care has powerful therapeutic effects on a range of physiological systems. This speeds up healing and maximizes recovery of the patient. Management of difficult aspects of care, such as pain during cancer, can be optimized with benefits to both patient and staff.

4. Communications provide a valuable therapeutic tool for patients who are incurable and maximizes their care. This increases the range of options for continued care in patients for whom cure is excluded, and provides an appropriate means of continuing input with such patients. Thus there is less justification for withdrawing from these patients.

5. Patients can be encouraged to have greater participation in decision making by using simple communication techniques. In so doing, patients are accepting greater responsibility for the final product. Because they have had a hand in determining that product, they have an interest in maintaining it. Therefore, there are good grounds to assume patients are more likely to maintain changes they helped to instigate in their lives. This applies to all age groups.

6. Improved communications are likely to result in greater staff satisfaction, with commensurate improvements in staff morale and retention. The benefits of this to the institution can be substantial.

7. It cannot be denied that staffing problems are real in most health care settings, and that time is limited. These are the most common reasons heard for why good communications cannot be implemented. However, this is more a problem of priorities. Very often, changes in the way things are done generate substantial change in outcomes. Thus, communications can be made a priority. This will require adaptation, but this in itself is not insurmountable.

8. By adopting an optimal style of care, communications care comes naturally. Once adopted, it is difficult to revert to older and more rigid task-oriented forms of care.

9. Once adopted, communications care leads to more holistic forms of care generally where feelings and attitudes are considered, and where treatment decisions are based on wider issues of life quality rather than solely biological activity.

For most of us the future is not high tech health but low tech individual responsibility. Most diseases affecting affluent countries are not curable, and are likely to remain that way for the (realistically) foreseeable future. Most treatments add only marginally to patients' lives; many detract substantially. Communication places the vehicle for change firmly in our hands. As long as people are encouraged to believe that someone else will fix things, there is no incentive to care for themselves. If people believe that there will always be a solution to problems, there is no incentive to change. Health care will not become more and more high tech. There is simply not enough money to provide high levels of care to everyone. Slowly, prevention will be emphasized and population-based measures are gradually being used to decide who gets access to the increasingly limited resources available.

People need to be encouraged to care for themselves and others within the networks of society that remain: their families (however constituted); their distributed work and social environments; their communities of mixed and changing groups. These are the systems that produce people, and the nature of these systems determines the nature of the people produced. The mutual nature of individuals within a social group defines both. If children are not given the opportunity to learn to take responsibility for their health and well-being, how can they be expected to do so as adults? It may appear overly optimistic that children could do this, but given opportunities, children learn without effort things that as adults we struggle to master (Montessori, 1978). Communications makes such developments possible.

However, before people can adopt greater responsibility they need access to information.

To adopt a communication-based health care model is to change the way we think about health and illness. Just as the sounds made by musical instruments have themselves no meaning, once orchestrated to a symphony they can move people to tears. So pain ceases to be simply an indication of tissue damage and becomes a process reflecting modes of suffering determined by the person's cultural, social and psychological context. Patients diagnosed as having a heart attack find their life and personal security fractured by the threat of death when they thought themselves young and healthy. Clearing an occluded artery does not clear an occluded life. All too often we lose sight of these points of view in contemporary practice.

Better communication care is the thin end of a wedge of change. Adopting a communications care approach will inevitably bring other changes to the practice of health care delivery. This should lead to a better quality of life for all concerned. To change the way we interact and practise health care can change the experience of illness and health for the patient and the practitioner. Eventually, a shift in practice and a shift in expectations can perhaps bring about a re-alignment in the sophistication and maturity of a population regarding their health.

Communications in most health service settings have a remarkably low priority; despite the central role of communications in health care, few health care educational programmes emphasize communication skills. Many assume that if people can talk, then they can deal with the many situations that often require a high degree of skill and sensitivity. Most medical schools now do include some communications training, the profession of medicine having been more thoroughly identified as having sometimes severe shortcomings in communications abilities. However, the priorities are still such that this training occupies one of the smallest fragments of a doctor's education, and only slightly more so of other groups such as nurses. This is all the more remarkable when we think that communications are the only aspect of professional skills that will be used with every patient seen.

References

Alexander DA and Ritchie E (1990). 'Stressors' and difficulties in dealing with the terminal patient. *J. Palliat Care*, 6: 28–33.

Alderson P (1993). *Children's Consent to Surgery*. Buckingham: Open University Press.

Alroy G, Ber R, Kramer D (1984). An evaluation of the short-term effects of an interpersonal skills course. *Med. Ed.*, 18:85–9.

Ahles TA, Blanchard EB, Ruckdeschel JC (1983). The multidimensional nature of cancer-related pain. *Pain*, 17: 277–88.

Anderson EA (1987). Preoperative preparation for cardiac surgery facilitates recovery, reduces psychological distress and reduces the incidence of acute postoperative hypertension. *J. Consult. Clin. Psychol.*, 55: 513–20.

Anderson RJ, Kirk LM (1982). Methods of improving patient compliance in chronic disease states, *Arch. Int. Med.*, 142: 1673–5.

Angell M (1984). Respecting the autonomy of competent patients. *N.E.J.M.*, 310: 1115–6.

Anisman H, Sklar LS (1984). Psychological insults and pathology. Contributions from neurochemical, hormonal and immunological mechanisms. In A Steptoe and A Mathews (Eds) *Health Care and Human Behaviour*. London: Academic Press.

Anthony S (1971). *The Discovery of Death in Childhood and After*. London: Allen-Lane.

Antoni MH, Goodkin K (1988). Host moderator variables in the promotion of cervical neoplasia: 1. Personality facets. *J. Psychosomat. Res.*, 32: 327–38.

Averill JR (1984). The acquisition of emotions during adulthood. In CZ Malatesta and CE Izard (Eds.) *Emotion in Adult Development*. Los Angeles: Sage.

Baddeley A (1986). *Working Memory*. Oxford: Clarendon.

Baile WR, DiMaggio JR, Schapira DV, Janofsky JS (1991). The request for assistance in dying. The need for psychiatric consultation. *Cancer*, 72: 2786–91.

Bakhai A, Goodman F, Juchniewichz H, Martin A., Porter G, White C, Williams L, Hopkins A (1990). How easy is it to contact the duty medical doctor responsible for acute admissions? *B.M.J.*, 301: 529–31.

Balk D (1983). Effect of sibling death on teenagers. *J. Pub. Health*, 53: 14–8.

Bande EB (1990). Children's coping with diabetes: Understanding the role of cognitive development. *J. Pediatr. Psychol.*, 15: 27–41.

Bandura A (1986). *Social Foundations of Thought and Action. A Social Cognitive Theory*. New Jessey: Prentice-Hall.

Bar-Tal D, Graumann CF, Kruglanski AW, Stroebe W (Eds.) (1989). *Sterotyping and Prejudice: Changing Conceptions*. New York: Springer-Verlag.

Bateson G (1973). *Steps to an Ecology of Mind*. St. Albans: Paladin.

Bainu C (1976). *Understanding Each Other*. San Francisco: Institute for General Semantics.

Beck AT, Emery G (1985). *Anxiety Disorders and Phobias in a Cognitive Perspective*. New York: Basic Books.

Becker MH, Maiman LA (1979) Sociobehavioural determinants of compliance with health care and medical recommendations. *Med. Care*, 13: 10–24.

Becker MH and Rosenstock IM (1984). Compliance with medical advice. In A Steptoe and A Mathews (Eds). *Health Care and Human Behaviour*. London: Academic Press.

Bedell SE, Delbanco TL (1984). Choices about cariopulmonary resuscitation in the hospital: When do physicians talk with patients? *N.E.J.M.*, 310, 1089–93.

Beecher HK (1946). Pain in men wounded in battle. *Anns. Surg.*, 123, 96–105.

Beecher HK (1961). Surgery as placebo: Quantitative study of bias. *J.A.M.A.*, 176, 1002–1007.

Benoliel JQ (1977). Nurses and the human experience of dying. In H Feifel (Ed) *New Meanings of Death*. New York: McGraw-Hill.

Ben Zira Z (1980). Affective and instrumental components in the physician patient relationship: An additional dimension in interaction theory. *J. Health Soc. Beh.*, 21: 170–80.

Bibace R, Walsh ME (1980). Development of children's conceptions of illness. *Paediatrics*, 66: 912–7.

Birdwhistell R (1970). *Kinesics and Context*. Harmondsworth: Penguin.

Blanchard C.G. and Ruckdeschel J.C. (1986). Psychosocial aspects of cancer in adults: implications for teaching medical students. J. Cancer Educ., 1, 237–248.

Blanchard CG, Labrecque MS, Ruckdeschel JC, Blanchard EB (1988). Information and decision-making preferences of hospitalized adult cancer patients. *Soc. Sci.Med.*, 27: 1139–45.

Black D (1986). *The Plague Years*. London: Picador.

Black RG (1975). The chronic pain syndrome. *Surg. Clinc. N.Amer.*, 55: 999–1011.

Blaxter M (1983). The causes of disease: Women talking. *Soc. Sci. Med.*, 17: 59–69.

Bluebond-Langener M (1978). *The Private World of the Dying Child*. Princeton: Princeton University Press.

Blumenhagen DW (1980). Hypertension: A folk illness with a medical name. *Cult., Med. Psychiat.*, 4: 197–227.

Bodmer WF, Cottrell S, Frischauf AM, Kerr IB, Murday VA, Rowan AJ, Smith MF, Solomon E, Thomas H and Varesco L (1989). Genetic analysis of colorectal cancer. *Proc. Int. Symposium Princess Takamatsu Cancer Res. Fund.* 20: 49–59.

Booth-Kewley S, Friedman HS (1987). Psychological predictors of heart disease: A quantative review. *Psych. Bull.*, 101: 343–62.

Bonica JJ (1984). Management of cancer pain. In M Zimmerman, P Drings and G Wagner (Eds), *Recent Results in Cancer Research*. Berlin: Springer.

Bowlby J (1978). *Attachment and Loss: Volume 2: Separation, Anxiety and Anger*. Harmondsworth: Penguin.

Bowlby J (1972). *Attachment and Loss: Volume 3: Loss, Sadness and Depression*. Harmondsworth: Penguin.

Boyle CM (1970). Difference between doctor's and patient's interpretations of some common medical terms. *B.M.J.*, 1 (704): 286–9.

Bradford R (1989). Obstacles to collaborative practice. *Nursing Manag.*, 20: 72i–72p.

Brewin TB (1991). Three ways of giving bad news. *Lancet*, 337: 1207–9.

Brewster AB (1982). Chronically ill hospitalised children's concepts of their illness. *Paediatrics*, 69: 609–15.

Brinkley D (1983). Emotional distress during cancer chemotherapy. *B.M.J.*, 286: 663–4.

Brody DS (1980a). The patient's role in clinical decision making. *Ann. Int. Med.*, 93: 718–22.

Brody DS (1980b). Physician recognition of behavioral, psychological and social aspects of medical care. *Arch. Int. Med.*, 140: 1286–9.

Broome ME, Bates TA, Lillis PP, McGahee TW (1990). Children's medical fears, coping behaviors, and pain perceptions during a lumbar puncture. *Oncol. Nurs. Forum.*, 117: 361–7.

Brown R, Kulik J (1982). Flashbulb memory. In U Neisser (Ed.) *Memory Observed*. New York: W.H. Freeman.

Brown JB, Weston WW, Stewart M (1991) Patient-centered interviewing part II: finding common ground. *Can. Fam. Physic.*, 35: 151–8.

Bryant LH, McFarland KF, Michels P (1990). The patient/physician relationship in the management of diabetes mellitus. *J. South Carolina Med. Assoc.*, 86: 389–91.

Buchan IC, Richardson IM (1973). Time study of consultations in general practice. *Scottish Health Studies* No. 27. Scottish Home and Health Department.

Buckalew LW, Salis R.E. (1986). Patient compliance and medication perception. *J.Clin.Psychol.*, 42: 49–53.

Buller MK, Buller DB (1987). Physicians' communication style and patient satisfaction. *J. Health Soc. Beh.*, 28: 375–88.

Burgess C, Morris T, Pettingale KW (1989). Psychological response to cancer diagnosis II. Evidence for coping styles (coping styles and cancer diagnosis). *J. Psychosom. Res.*, 32: 263–72.

Burroughs J, Hoffbrand B. (1990). A critical look at nursing observations. *Postgrad. Med. J.*, 66: 370–72.

Byrne PS, Long BEL (1976). *Doctors Talking to Patients*. London: H.M.S.O.

Candy CE (1991). 'Not for resuscitation': the student nurses' viewpoint. *J. Adv. Nurs.*, 16: 138–46.

Carey WB (1969). Psychological sequelea of early infancy health crisis. *Clin. Paediat.*, 8: 459–63.

Carmel S, Bernstein J (1986). Identifying with the patient: and intensive programme for medical students. *Med. Ed.*, 20: 432–6.

Carmi R (1991). Genetic counselling to a traditional society *Lancet*, 337: 306.

Carnevale FA (1990). A description of stressors and coping strategies among parents of critically ill children — a preliminary study. *Intensive Care Nurs.*, 6: 4–11.

Carr EC (1990). Postoperative pain: patients' expectations and experiences. *J. Adv. Nurs.*, 15: 89–100.

Cartwright A (1964). *Human Relations and Hospital Care*. London: Routledge and Keegan Paul.

Cartwright A, Hockey L, Anderson JL (1973). *Life Before Death*. London: Routledge and Kegan Paul.

Cartwright A, O'Brien M (1978). Social class variations in health care and the nature of general practice communications. In D Tuckett and JM Kaufert (Eds) B*asic Readings in Medical Sociology*, London: Tavistock.

Cartwright PD (1985). Pain control after surgery: A survey of current practice. *Ann. R. Coll. Surg. Engl.*, 67: 13–6.

Cassell EJ (1982). The nature of suffering and the goals of medicine. *N.E.J.M.*, 306: 639–45.

Cassem NH, Hackett TP (1971). Psychiatric consultation in a coronary care unit. *Ann. Intern. Med.*, 75: 9–14.

Cerkoney AB, Hart K (1980). The relationship between the health belief model and compliance of persons with diabetes mellitus. *Diabetes Care,* 3: 594–8.

Christine-Seeley J (1981). Preventive medicine and the family. *Can. Fam. Phys.*, 27: 449–55.

Cicourel A (1975). Discourse and text: cognitive and linguistic processes in studies of social structure. Versus: Quaderni di Studi Semiotica, Sept. Dec: 33–84.

Cicourel A (1978). Language and society: Cognitive, cultural and linguistic aspects of language use. *Sozialwissenschaftliche Annalen*, 2: 25–58.

Cicourel A (1980). Three models of discourse analysis: The role of social structure. *Discourse Processes*, 3: 101–32.

Clarke A (1991) Is non-directive genetic counselling possible? *Lancet,* 338: 998–1001.

Cleeland CS (1987a). Barriers to the management of cancer pain. *Oncology,* 1 (2 Suppl), 19–26.

Cleeland CS (1987b). Non-pharmacological management of cancer pain. *J. Pain Sympt. Manage.*, 1, 209–15.

Coghill SR, Caplan HL, Alexandra H, Robson KM, Kumar R (1986). Impact of maternal post-natal depression on cognitive development of young children. *B.M.J.*, 292: 1165–7.

Cohen G, Eysenk M, LeVoi ME (1986). *Memory: A Cognitive Approach*. Milton Keynes: Open University Press.

Cousins N (1979). *Anatomy of an Illness: As Perceived by the Patient. Reflections on Healing and Regeneration*. New York: WW Norton and Co.

Cox JL, Connor Y, Kendell RE (1982). Prospective study of the psychiatric disorders of childbirth. *Br. J. Psychiat.*, 140: 111–7.

Craig KD (1986). Social modeling influences: Pain in context. In RA Sternbach (Ed) T*he Psychology of Pain*. New York: Raven Press.

Craik FIM, Lockhart RS (1972). Levels of processing: a framework for memory research. *J. Verbal Learn. Verb. Beh.*, 11: 671–84.

Darwin C (1972). The Expression of Emotions in Man and Animals. London: John Murray (1965. Chicago: University of Chicago Press).

Davis CL, Hardy JR (1994). Palliative care. *B.M.J.*, 308: 1359–62.

Davis DL, Stewart M, Harmon RJ (1989). Postponing pregnancy after perinatal death: Perspectives on doctor advice. *Ann. Am. Acad. Child Adolesc. Psychiatry*, 8: 481–7.

Delvaux N, Razavi D, Farvacques C (1988). Cancer care — A stress for health professionals. *Soc. Sci. Med.*, 27: 159–66.

Derogatis RL (1986a). The unique impact of breast and gynaecological cancers on body image and sexual identity in women. In JM Vaeth (Ed) *Body Image, Self-Esteem and Sexuality in Cancer Patients* (2nd Ed). Basle: Karger.

Derogatis LR (1986b). Psychology in cancer medicine: A perspective and overview. *J. Consult. Clin. Psychol.*, 54: 632–8.

Dozor RB, Meece KS (1990). Relationships with AIDS patients: Clinical metaphors and preventive bioethics. *Fam-Med.*, 22: 474–7.

Drass KA (1982). Negotiation and the structure of discourse in medical consultation. *Sociol. Health Ill.*, 4: 320–41.

D'Saint-Exupery A (1942). *Night Flight/Southern Mail*. Harmondsworth: Penguin Classics.

Eagly AH, Ashmore RD, Makhijani MG, Longro LC (1991) What is beautiful is good, but . . . : A meta-analytic review of research on the physical attractiveness sterotype. *Psych. Bull.*, 110: 109–28.

Egbert L, Battit G, Welch C, Bartlett M (1964). Reduction of post-operative pain by encouragment and instruction of patients. *N.E.J.M.*, 270: 825–7.

Eisenthal S, Emery R, Lazare A, Udin H (1982). Adherence and the negotiated approach to patienthood. *Arch. Gen. Psychiat.*, 36: 393–8.

Eiser C (1984). Communicating with sick and hospitalised children. *J. Child Psychol. and Psychiat.*, 25: 181–9.

Ekman P (1972). Universals and cultural differences in facial expressions of emotions. Current Theory and Research in Motivation. Nebraska Symposium on Motivation, Vol XIX, 207–83.

Ellis A (1970). *The Essence of Rational Psychotherapy*. New York: Institute For Rational Living.

Erikson EH (1963). *Childhood and Society* (2nd Ed). New York: Norton.

Ettinger DS (1986). The clinical use of anti-emetics. In RL Derogatis (Ed) *Clinical Psychopharmacology*. Menlo Park, Ca: Addison-Wesley.

Evans BJ, Kiellerup FD, Stanley RO, Burrows GD, Sweet B (1987). A communication skills programme for increasing patients' satisfaction with general practice consultation. *Br. J. Med. Psychol.*, 60: 373–8.

Eysenk M (1986). Working memory. In G Cohen, M Eysenk and ME

LeVoi (Eds) *Memory: A Cognitive Approach*. Milton Keynes: Open University Press.

Field D (1984). Formal instruction in United Kingdom medical schools about death and dying. *Med. Ed.*, 18: 429–34.

Field D (1989). Nurse's accounts of nursing the terminally ill on a coronary care unit. *Intensive Care Nurs.*, 5: 114–22.

Fielding R (1984). *An Investigation into the Role of Psychological Factors During Recovery from Myocardial Infarction*. Unpublished Doctoral Thesis, University of Sheffield, U.K.

Fielding R (1987). Patients' beliefs regarding the causes of myocardial infarction: Implications for information giving and compliance. *Pat. Ed. Counsel.*, 9: 121–34.

Fielding R (1989). Cognition, control and mood during recovery from AMI, Abstracts of International Conference of Health Psychology, 23 September, Cardiff. B.P.S.

Fielding R,Tam FSH (1989). Role and context in the perception of distress. *Bull. Hong Kong Psychol. Soc.*, 22/23: 29–43.

Fielding R (1991). Depression and acute myocardial infarction: A review and reinterpretation. *Soc. Sci. and Med.*, 32: 1017–27.

Fielding R, Wong DKN, Ong SG (1992) Symptoms, blood-pressure information and mood effects on symptom recall. *Psychology and Health*, 7: 323–30.

Fielding R, Lo A, Cheng KK, Pei GK, Hedley AJ, Pang KH, Mak KH, Shung E (1990). Doctor shopping behaviour in a southern Chinese urban community. Manuscript published by Department of Community Medicine and Unit for Behavioural Science, University of Hong Kong.

Fielding R (1994). Discrepencies between patient and nurse perceptions of post-operative pain: Shortcomings in pain control. *J.Hong Kong. Med. Assoc.*, 46: 142–6.

Fielding R, Ko L, Wong LSW (1995). Inconsistencies between belief and practice: Assessment of Chinese cancer patients' knowledge of their disease. *J. Cancer Care*, 4: 11–5.

Fielding R, Ko L, Wong L, Hedley A.J, Gilhooly MLM, Tam FSH (1994). Prevalence and determinants of diagnostic and prognostic disclosure by radiotherapists and surgeons to patients with terminal cancer in Hong Kong. *J. Hong Kong Med. Assoc.*, 46: 220–230.

Finlay I, Dallimore D (1991). Your child is dead. *B.M.J.*, 302: 1524–5.

Fishman B, Loscalzo M (1987). Cognitive-behavioural interventions in management of cancer pain: Principles and applications. *Med. Clin. N. Amer.*, 71: 271–87.

Foley GV, McCarthy AM (1976). The child with leukemia in a special haematology clinic. *Am J. Nurse.* 76: 1115–9.

Foley KM (1985). The treatment of cancer pain. *N.E.J.M.*, 313: 84–9.

Foley KM (1986). The clinical use of analgesics. In RL Derogatis (Ed) *Clinical Psychopharmacology*. Menlo Park, Ca: Addison-Wesley.

Fordyce WE (1976). *Behavioural Methods for Chronic Pain and Illness*. St. Louis: Moseby.

Fraley AM (1990). Chronic sorrow: A parental response. *J. Pediat. Nurs.*, 5: 268–73.

Francis V, Korsch BM, Morris MJ (1969). Gaps in doctor-patient communication: patients' response to medical advice. *N.E.J.M.*, 280: 535–40.

French K (1979). Some anxieties of elective surgery patients and the desire for reassurance and information. In DJ Oborne, MM Gruneberg and JR Eiser (Eds) *Research in Psychology and Medicine* Vol. I. London: Academic.

Freeling P (1986). Communication between doctors and nurses. In J Walton and G. McLachlan (Eds) *Partnership or Prejudice: Communication Between Doctors and Those in the Other Caring Professions*. London: Nuffield Provincial Hospitals Trust.

Friedson E (1961). *Patients' Views of Medical Practice*. New York: Russell Sage Foundation.

Friedson E (1970a). *Profession of Medicine*. New York: Harper and Row.

Friedson E (1970b). *Professional Dominance*. Chicago: Atherton Press.

Friedman SB, Chodoff P, Mason JW (1963). Behavioural observations of parents anticipating the death of a child. *Paediats.*, 32: 610–25.

Frijda NH (1986). *The Emotions*. Paris: Cambridge University Press.

Frisby JP (1986). The computational approach to vision. In I Roth and JP Frisby (Ed) *Perception and Representation: A Cognitive Approach*. Milton Keynes: Open University Press.

Fry PS (1990). A factor analytic investigation of home-bound elderly individuals' concerns about death and dying, and their coping responses. *J. Clin. Psychol.*, 46: 737–48.

Gilbooly MLM, Berkeley JS, McCann K, Gibling F, Murray K (1988). Truth telling with dying cancer patients. *Palliative Med.*, 2: 64–71.

Glaser BG, Strauss AL (1965). *Awareness of Dying*. Chicago: University of Chicago Press.

Goldberg DP, Blackwell B (1970). Psychiatric illness in general practice:a detailed study using new methods of case identification. *B.M.J.*, 270: 439–42.

Gordon DR (1990). Embodying illness, embodying cancer. *Cult. Med. Psychiatry*, 14: 275–97.

Greer S, Morris T, Pettingale KW (1979). Psychological response to breast cancer: Effect on outcome. *Lancet*, ii: 785–7.

Gunnell D, Frankel S (1994). Prevention of suicide: Aspirations and evidence. *B.M.J.*, 308: 1227–33.

Gutton P (1978). Psychopathology of the physically sick child. *Revue Neuropsychiat. Infant.*, 26: 471–6.

Hamilton SC (1987). *A Communications Audit Handbook: Helping Organizations Communicate.* London: Longman.

Hampton JR, Harrison MJG, Mitchell JRA, Pritchard JS, Seymour C (1975). Relative contributions of history taking, physical examination, and laboratory investigation to diagnosis and management of medical outpatients. *B.M.J.*, 277: 486–9.

Hanratty P (1983). Care of the dying patient. *J. Royal Soc. Health*, 103: 1–4.

Harre R, Clarke D, De Carlo N (1984). *Motives and Mechanisms.* London: Methuen.

Hart SK, Moore MN (1989). The relationship among organizational climate variable and nurse stability in critical care units. *J. Prof. Nurs.*, 5: 124–31.

Hart-Zeldin C, Kalnins IV, Pollack P, Love R (1990). Children in the context of ' Achieving Health for All: a Framework for Health Promotion'. *Can. J. Public Health*, 81: 196–8.

Havik OE, Maeland JG (1986). Verbal denial and outcome of myocardial infarction patients. *J. Psychosomat. Res.*, 32: 145–57.

Hawkins C, Paterson I (1987). Medicolegal audit in the West Midlands region: Analysis of 100 cases. *B.M.J.*, 295: 1533–6.

Heberden W (1872). Some account of a disorder of the breast. *Med. Transact. Coll. Physicians* (London), 2: 59–67.

Heiney SP, Goon-Johnson K, Ettinger RS, Ettinger S (1990). The effects of group therapy on siblings of pediatric oncology patients. *J. Pediatr. Oncol. Nurs.*, 7: 95–100.

Herriot P (1974). *Attributes of Memory.* London: Methuen.

Herth K (1990). Fostering hope in terminally-ill people. *J. Adv. Nurs.*, 15: 1250–9.

Hiew TM, Lim KW (1990). Cockayne's syndrome — Difficulties with early diagnosis. *Singapore Med. J.*, 31: 558–63.

High DM (1989). Truth telling, confidentiality, and the dying patient: New dilemmas for the nurse. *Nurs-Forum.* 24: 5–10.

Hill HF, Saeger LC, Chapman CR (1986). Patient controlled analgesia after bone marrow transplantation for cancer. *Postgrad. Med.*, August: 33–40.

Hinton J (1972). *Dying.* Harmondsworth: Penguin.

Hobson B (1984). *Forms of Feeling: The art of Psychotherapy.* London: Tavistock.

Hogbin B, Fallowfield L (1989). Getting it taped: The 'bad news' consultation with cancer patients. *Br. J. Hospital Med.*, 41: 330–3.

Holdaway J (1985). The management of dying patients in New Zealand coronary care units. *N.Z. Med. J*, 98: 639–41.

Houghton H (1968). Problems in hospital communication. In G McClachlan (Ed) *Problems and Progress in Medical Care*. London: Nuffield.

Howie JGR, Bigg AR (1980). Family trends in psychotropic and antibiotic prescribing in general practice. *B.M.J.*, 286: 836–8.

Hughes S, Henley A (1990). *Dealing with Death in Hospital: Procedures for Managers and Staff*. London: King Edward's Hospital Fund.

Issel LM, Ersek M, Lewis FM (1990). How children cope with mother's breast cancer. *Oncol. Nurs. Forum*, 17 (3 Suppl): 5–12.

Jacobson AM., Hauser ST, Lavori P, Wolfsdorf JI, Herskowitz RD, Milley JE, Bliss R, Gelfand E, Wertlieb D, Stein J (1990). Adherence among children and adolescents with insulin-dependent diabetes mellitus over a four-year longitudinal follow-up: I. The influence of patient coping and adjustment. *J. Pediatr. Psychol.*, 15: 511–26.

James I, Milne DL, Firth H (1990). A systematic comparison of feedback and staff discussion in changing the ward atmosphere. *J. Adv. Nurs.*, 15: 329–36.

Janis I (1958). *Psychological Stress*. New York: Wiley.

Janson S, Jayakoddy A, Abulaban A, Gustavson KH (1991). Severe mental retardation in Jordanian children. A retrospective study. *Acta. Paediatr. Scand.*, 79: 1099–104.

Jaruzelska J, Henriksen KF, Guttler F, Riess O, Borski K, Blin N, Slomski R (1991). The codon 408 mutation associated with haplotype 2 is predominant in Polish families with phenylketonuria. *Hum. Genet.*, 86: 247–50.

Jay SM, Elliott CH, Ozolons M, Olson RA, Pruitt SD (1985). Behavioural management of children's distress during painful medical procedures. *Beh Res. Ther.*, 23: 513–20.

Jeffery P, Lansdown R (1982). The role of the special school in the care of the dying child. *Dev. Med. Child Neurol.*, 24: 693–7.

Jones DA, Vetter NJ (1984). A survey of those who care for the elderly at home: their problems and their needs. *Soc. Sci. Med.*, 19: 511–5.

Kahneman D, Slovic P, Tversky A (1984). *Judgement Under Uncertainty: Heuristics and Biases*. Cambridge: Cambridge University Press.

Kalish RA (1966). Social distance and the dying. *Commun. Ment. Health. J.*, 2: 152–9.

Kane B (1979). Children's concepts of death. *J. Genetic Psych.*, 134: 141–53.

Kastenbaum R (1974). Childhood: The kingdom where creatures die. *J. Clin. Child Psychol.*, 3: 11–4.

Keele SW, Neill WT (1978). Mechanisms of attention. In EC Carterette and MP Friedman (Eds) *Handbook of Perception*, Vol. IX. London: Academic Press.

Kessel N (1986). Communication between doctors and social workers. In J Walton and G. McLachlan (Eds) *Partnership or Prejudice: Communication Between Doctors and Those in the Other Caring Professions.* London: Nuffield Provincial Hospitals Trust.

Kiecolt-Glaser JK, Glaser R, Strain EC, Stout JC, Tarr KL, Holliday JE, Speicher CE (1986). Modulation of cellular immunity in medical students. *J. Beh. Med.*, 9: 5–23.

Knudson GG, Natterson JA (1960). Participation of parents in the hospital care of fatally ill children. *Paediat.*, 26: 482.

Korsch BM, Gozzi EK, Francis V (1968). Gaps in doctor-patient communication: 1. doctor patient interaction and patient satisfaction. *Paediat.*, 42: 855–71.

Korsch BM, Negrete VF (1972). Doctor-patient communication. *Scientific American*, August: 66–73.

Kotarba JA (1983). Perceptions of death, belief systems and the process of coping with chronic pain. *Soc. Sci. Med.*, 17: 681–9.

Krulik T (1987). Loneliness and social isolation in school-age children with chronic life-threatening illness. In T Krulik, B Holaday and IM Martinson (Eds) *The Child and Family Facing Life-threatening Illness.* Philadelphia: J.B. Lippincott Co.

Lademann A (1987) The neurologically handicapped child. *Scand. Audiol. Supp.*, 10: 23–26.

Lamerton R (1973). *Care of the Dying.* Harmondsworth: Penguin.

Larkin H (1988). Communication can prevent med staff conflict. *Hospitals*, March 20: 109.

LaMontagne LL (1987). Factors influencing children's reactions and adjustment to illness: Implications for facilitating coping. In T Krulik, B Holaday and IM Martinson (Eds) *The Child and Family Facing Life-threatening Illness.* Philadelphia: J.B. Lippincott Co.

LaMontagne LL, Pawlak R (1990). Stress and coping of parents of children in a pediatric intensive care unit. *Heart and Lung*, 19: 416–21.

Lanes SF (1988). The logic of causal inference in medicine. In KJ Rothman (Ed) *Causal Inference.* Boston: Epidemiology Resources Inc.

Laron Z, Galatzer A, Amir S, Gil R, Karp M (1989). Psycho-social aspects of children and adolescents with diabetes. *Indian J. Pediat.*, 56, Suppl 1: 129–32.

Lazarus RL (1966). *Psychological Stress and the Coping Process.* New York: McGraw-Hill.

Lazarus RS, Launier R (1978). Stress-related transactions between person and environment. In LA Pervin and M Lewis (Eds) *Perspectives in Interactional Psychology.* New York: Plenum Press.

LeBaron S and Zelter LK (1985). The role of imagery in the treatment of dying children and adolescents. *J. Dev. Behav. Pediatr.*, 6: 252–8.

Levin DN, Cleeland CS, Dar R (1985). Public attitudes towards cancer pain. *Cancer,* 56: 2337–9.

Leonard I, Babbs C, Creed F (1990). Psychiatric referrals within the hospital — the communication process. *J. R. Soc. Med.,* 83: 241–4.

Levine J, Warrenberg S, Kerns R, Schwartz G, Delaney R, Fontana A, Gradman A, Smith S, Allen S, Cascione R (1987). The role of denial in recovery from coronary heart disease. *Psychosomat. Med.,* 49: 109–17.

Levy MH (1987/1988). Pain control research in the terminally ill. *Omega,* 18: 265–79.

Lewis FM, Woods NF, Hough EE, Bensley LS (1989). The family's functioning with chronic illness in the mother: the spouse's perspective. *Soc. Sci. Med.,* 29: 1261–9.

Lewis CE, Lewis MA, Lorimer MPH, Palmer BP (1977). Child initiated care: The use of school nursing services by children in an 'adult-free' system. *Paediat.,* 60: 499–507.

Lewis MA, Lewis CE (1990). Consequences of empowering children to care for themselves. *Pediat.,* 17(2): 63–7.

Ley P (1972). Complaints made by hospital staff and patients: A review of the literature. *Bull. Br. Psych. Soc.,* 115–20.

Ley P, Bradshaw PW, Eaves DE, Walker CM (1973). A method for increasing patients' recall of information presented to them. *Psychol. Med.,* 3: 217–20.

Ley P, Spelman MS (1972). *Communicating With the Patient.* London: Staples.

Ley P (1977). Doctor-patient communication. In S Rachman (Ed) *Contributions to Medical Psychology,* Vol. I. Oxford: Pergamon.

Littlewood R (1991). From disease to illness and back again. *Lancet,* 337: 1013–6.

Lo AY, Hedley AJ, Pei GK, Ong SG, Ho LM, Fielding R, Cheng KK, Daniel L (1994). Doctor shopping in Hong Kong: Implications for quality assurance. *Int. J. Qual Health Care,* 6: 371–81.

Lutz CA (1988). *Unnatural Emotions.* Chicago: University of Chicago Press.

Macaskill S, MacDonald MB (1982). Childhood 5–10: An exploratory study of parental experience. Research Report of Department of Marketing, University of Strathclyde, Glasgow.

Maclure A, Stewart GT (1984). Admission of children to hospital in Glasgow: Relation to unemployment and other deprivation variables. *Lancet,* 22/9: 682–5.

Maguire GP, Julier DL, Hawton KE, Bancroft JHJ (1974). Psychiatric morbidity and referral on two general medical wards. *B.M.J.,* 276: 266.

Maguire P (1984a). Communication skills and patient care. In A Steptoe and A Mathews (Eds) Health Care and Human Behaviour. London: Academic Press.

Maguire P (1984b). Affective disorder in cancer patients. *Int. Rev. Applied. Psychol.*, 33: 479–91.

Maguire P (1985). Barriers to the psychological care of the dying. *B.M.J.*, 291: 1711–3.

Maguire P, Faulkner A (1988). Communicating with cancer patients: I. Handling bad news and difficult questions. *B.M.J.*, 297: 907–9.

Marks JN, Goldberg DP, Hillier V (1979). Determinants of the ability of general practitioners to detect psychiatric illness. *Psycholog. Med.*, 9: 337–53.

Martin TO (1982). Death anxiety and social desirability among nurses. *Omega*, 13: 51–7.

Martineau TM (1989) Psychological costs of screening. *B.M.J.*, 299: 527.

Maslow AH (1954). *Motivation and Personality* (2nd Ed). New York: Harper and Row.

Mason JW (1968). A review of psychoendocrine research on the pituitary-adrenal cortical system. *Psychosomat. Med.*, 30: 567–607.

Massey JA, Reimels EM (1986). Failure to collaborate? *J. Prof. Nurs.*, 2: 276.

Matthews A, Ridgeway V (1984). Preparation for surgery. In A Steptoe and A Mathews (Eds) Health Care and Human Behaviour. London: Academic Press.

McGhee SM (1990). Structured medical records and clinical protocols: A systematic approach to patient management. *Proc. First Hong Kong Medical Informatics Conference*: 3–7.

McIntee J, Firth H (1984). How to beat the burn out. *Health and Soc. Serv. J.*, Feb. 9: 166–8.

McKeown T (1976). *The Role of Medicine: Dream, Mirage or Nemesis.* Oxford: Nuffield Provincial Hospitals Trust.

McMahon R (1990). Power and collegial relations among nurses on wards adopting primary nursing and hierarchical ward management structures. *J Adv Nurs*, 15: 32–9.

Mechanic D (1962). The concept of illness behaviour. *J. Chron. Dis.*, 15: 189–94.

Melzack R, Wall PD (1982) *The Challenge of Pain.* Harmondsworth: Penguin.

Merskey H (1986). Classification of chronic pain: Descriptions of chronic pain syndromes and definitions of pain terms. *Pain*, Suppl. 3: s1–226.

Meyer DL, Leventhal H Gutman M (1985). Common-sense models of illness: The example of hypertension. *Health Psychology*, 4: 115–35.

Michembaum D, Turk D (1987). *Facilitating Treatment Adherence.* New York: Plenum.

Mikail SF, von Baeyer CL (1990). Pain, somatic focus, and emotional adjustment in children of chronic headache sufferers and controls. *Soc. Sci. Med*, 31: 51–9.

Miller FJW, Court WDM, Walton WS, Knox EG (1960). *Growing up in Newcastle-On-Tyne*. London: Oxford University Press.

Miller SM (1987). Monitoring and blunting: validation of a questionnaire to assess styles of information seeking under threat. *J. Person. Soc. Psychol*, 52: 345–53.

Montessori M (1978). *The Secret of Childhood*. (Translation by B Barclay-Carter.) India: Orient Longman.

Morris T, Greer S, Watson M, Pettingale KW(1981). Patterns of expression of anger and their psychological correlates in women with breast caner. *J. Psychosomat. Med.*, 25: 111–7.

Murphy T (1973). Cancer pain. *Postgrad. Med.*, 53: 187–94.

Narod S (1991). Counselling under genetic heterogeneity: A practical approach. *Clin. Genet.*, 31: 125–31.

Natterson JA, Knudson GG (1960). Observations concerning the fear of death in fatally ill children and their mothers. *Psychosomat. Med.*, 22: 456–65.

Nerenz D, Leventhal H (1983). Self-regulation theory in chronic illness. In TG Burish and L Bradley (Eds) *Coping With Chronic Illness: Research and Applications*. New York: Academic Press.

Nerenz DR, Leventhal H, Love RR, Ringler KE (1984). Psychological aspects of cancer chemotherapy. *Int. Rev. Applied Psychol.*, 33: 521–9.

Ng SKC (1991). Does epidemiology need a new philosophy? A case study of logical enquiry in the Acquired Immunodeficiency Syndrome. *Am J. Epidemiol.*, 133: 1073–7.

Norman DA, Shallice T (1980) Attention to action. Willed and automatic control of behaviour. University of California San Diego CHIP Report 99.

O'Connor DW, Pollitt PA, Treasure FP, Brook CPB, Reiss BB (1989). The influence of education, social class and sex on Mini-Mental State scores. *Psycholog. Med.*, 19: 771–6.

O'Hara MW, Ghoneim MM, Hinrichs JV, Mehta MP, Wright EJ (1989). Psychosocial consequences of surgery. *Psychosomat. Med.*, 51: 356–70.

Onadim Z, Hykin PG, Hungerford JL, Cowell JK (1991). Genetic counselling in retinoblastoma: importance of ocular fundus examination of first degree relatives and linkage analysis. *Br. J. Ophthalmol.*, 75: 147–50.

OPCS: Office of Population Censuses and Surveys (1989). *Women's Experience of Maternity Care — A Postal Survey Manual*. London: HMSO.

Ormel J, Van Den Brink W, Koeter MWJ, Giel R, Van Der Meer K, Van De Wilige G, Wilmink FW (1990). Recognition, management and outcome of psychological disorders in primary care: A naturalistic follow-up study. *Psych. Med.*, 20: 909–23.

Palmer PES (1985). The epidemic of investigations. *Int. J. Epidemiol.*, 14: 359–62.

Parkes KR (1984). Locus of control, cognitive appraisal and coping in stressful episodes. *J. Pers. Soc. Psychol.*, 46: 655–68.

Parkes CM (1972). *Bereavement: Studies of Grief in Adult Life*. Harmondsworth. Penguin.

Parkes CM (1985). Bereavement. *B.J. Psychiat.*, 146: 11–7.

Pasacreta JV, Jacobsen PB (1989). Addressing the need for staff support among nurse caring for the AIDS population. *Oncol Nurs Forum*, 16: 659–63.

Pennebaker JW (1982) *The Psychology of Physical Symptoms*. New York: Springer.

Perlin L, Schooner C (1978). The structure of coping. *J. Health Soc. Beh.*, 19: 2–21.

Perrin EC, Gerrity PS (1981). There's a demon in your belly: Children's understanding of illness. *Paediatrics*, 67: 841–9.

Petermann F, Bode U (1986). Five coping styles in families of children with cancer: a retrospective study in thirty families. *Pediatr. Hematol. Oncol.*, 3: 299–309.

Podell RN (1975). *A Physician's Guide to Compliance in Hypertension*. Rahway, New Jersey: Merck.

Pratt JW, Mason A (1984). The meaning of touch in care practice. *Soc. Sci. Med.*, 18: 1081–8.

Price TR, Bergen BJ (1977). The relationship to death as a source of stress for nurses on a coronary care unit. *Omega*, 8: 229–37.

Querido A (1967). *The Efficiency of Medical Care*. Leiden: Steufert- Kroese.

Rahe RH (1989). Paper presented to the Victoria College of Psychiatrists, Melbourne, Australia, June 1989.

Ramirez AJ, Craig TKJ, Watson JP, Fentiman IS, North WRS, Rubens RD (1989). Stress and relapsed breast cancer. *B.M.J.*, 294: 291–3.

Ray C (1991). Chronic fatigue syndrome and depression: Conceptual and methodological ambiguities. *Psycholog. Med.*, 21: 1–9.

Reed SB (1990). Potential for alterations in family process: When a family has a child with cystic fibrosis. *Issues Compr. Pediatr. Nurs.*, 13: 15–23.

Revans RW (1964). *Standards for Morale: Cause and Effect in Hospitals*. London: Oxford University Press.

Reynolds PM, Sanson-Fisher KW, Poole AD, Harker J (1984). Cancer and communication: Information giving in the oncology clinic. *B.M.J.*, 282: 449–51.

Rich CL, Warstadt GM, Nemiroff RA, Fowler KC, Warstadt GM (1991). Suicide, stressors and the life cycle. *Am. J. Psychiat.*, 48: 524–7.

Richards MPM (1974). The first steps to becoming social. In MPM Richards (Ed) *The Integration of a Child into a Social World.* Cambridge: Cambridge University Press.

Ritchie JA, Caty S, Ellerton ML (1988). Coping behaviors of hospitalized preschool children. *Matern. Child. Nurs. J.*, 17: 153–71.

Rothstein P (1980). Psychological stress in families of children in a paediatric intensive care unit. *Paediat. Clin. N.Am.*, 27: 613–20.

Rousseau P (1988). Perinatal bereavement. Psychopathology and counseling. *J. Gynecol. Obstet. Biol. Reprod. Paris,* 17: 285–94.

Rutter M (1979). Stress, coping and development: some issues and some questions. *J. Child Psychol. Psychiat.*, 22: 323–56.

Sackett DL (1976). Magnitude of compliance and non-compliance. In DL Sackett and RP Haynes (Eds) *Compliance With Medical Regimens.* Baltimore: Johns Hopkins University Press.

Schacter S (1971). *Emotion, Obesity and Crime.* New York: Academic Press.

Schain WS (1990). Physician-patient communication about breast cancer. A challenge for the 1990s. *Surg. Clin. North. Am.*, 70: 917–36.

Schulman BA (1979). Active patient orientation and outcomes in hypertensive treatment. *Medical Care,* 17: 267–80.

Schultz R, Anderman D (1979). Physicians' death anxiety and patient outcomes. *Omega,* 9: 327–32.

Scott N, Weiner MF (1984). 'Patientspeak': An exercise in communication. *J. Med. Ed.,* 59 890–3.

Seigel S (1975). Evidence from rats that morphine tolerance is a learned response. *J. Comparative Physiolog. Psychol.*, 89: 498–506.

Seigle S (1977). Morphine tolerance acquisition as an associative process. *Experi. Psychol. Animal Beh. Process,* 3: 1–13.

Seligman MEP (1975) *Helplessness: On Depression, Development and Death.* San Francisco: Freeman.

Seto WH, Ching PT, Fung JP, Fielding R (1989). The role of communication in the alteration of patient-care practices in hospital — A prospective study. *J. Hosp Infect ,* 14: 29–37.

Shapiro J (1983). Family reactions and coping strategies in response to the physically ill or handicapped child: A review. *Soc. Sci. Med.*, 17: 913–31.

Shield JPH, Baum JD (1994). Children's consent to treatment. *B.M.J.*, 308: 1182–3

Simpson M, Buckman R, Stewart M, Maguire P, Lipkin M, Novack D, Till J (1991). Doctor-patient communication: The Toronto consensus statement. *B.M.J.*, 303: 1385–7.

Sinclair J, Coulthard R (1975). *Towards and Analysis of Discourse*. New York: Oxford University Press.

Skipper J, Leonard RC (1978). Children, stress and hospitalization. In D Tuckett and JM Kaufert (Eds) Basic Readings in Medical Sociology, London: Tavistock.

Spicker SF, Ratzan RM (1990). Ars medicina et conditio humana. Edmund D. Pellegrino, M.D., on his 70th birthday. *J. Med. Philos*. 15: 327–41.

Sontag S (1977). *Illness as Metaphore*. Harmondsworth: Penguin.

Speece MW, Brent SB (1988). Childrens' understanding of death: a review of three components of a death concept. In T Krulik, B Holaday and IM Martinson (Eds) *The Child and Family Facing Life-threatening Illness*. Philadelphia: J.B. Lippincott Co.

Spelman MS, Ley P (1966). Knowledge of lung cancer and smoking habits. *Br. J. Soc. Clin. Psychol.*, 5: 207–10.

Spelman MS, Ley P, Jones CC (1966). How do we improve doctor-patient communications in our hospitals? *World Hospitals*, 2: 126–9.

Solomon GF (1981). Emotional and personality factors in the onset and course of autoimmune disease, particularly rheumatoid arthritis. In A Ader (Ed) *Psychoneuroimmunology*. New York: Academic Press.

Starr TJ, Pearlman RA, Uhlmann RF (1986). Quality of life and resuscitation decisions in elderly patients. *J. Gen. Intern. Med.*, 1: 373–9.

Sternbach RA (1976). Psychological factors in pain. In JJ Bonica and D Albe-Fessard (Eds) *Advances in Pain research and Therapy* (Vol. 1). New York: Raven Press.

Strand E (1979). Living with a handicapped child: How can we face the strain. *N.Z. Nurs. J.*, April: 30–32.

Sundaresan N, DiGiancinto GV (1988). Antitumour and antinocioceptive approaches to control cancer pain. *Med. Clin. N. Amer.*, 71: 329–48.

Sweeting HN, Gilhooly MLM (1990). Anticipatory grief: A review. *Soc. Sci. Med.*, 30: 1073–80.

Swenson-Feldman E, Brugge-Wiger P (1985). Promotion of interdisciplinary practice through an automated information system. *ANS*, 7: 39–47.

Szasz T, Hollender M (1965). A contribution to the philosophy of medicine: the basic models of the doctor-patient relationship. *Arch. Int. Med.*, 97: 585.

Taylor CM, Crisler JR (1988). Concerns of persons with cancer as perceived by cancer patients, physicians, and rehabilitation counsellors. *J. Rehabilit.*, January-March: 23–28.

Taylor SC (1980). Siblings need a plan of care too. *Paediat. Nurs.*, Nov/Dec: 9–13.

Teasdale JD, Barnard PJ (1993). *Affect, Cognition and Change: Remodelling Depressive Thought*. Hove: Lawrence Erlbaum Associates.

Tebbi CK, Cummings KM, Zevon MA, Smith L, Richards M, Mallon J (1986). Compliance of paediatric and adolescent cancer patients. *Health Psychol.*, 3: 553–62.

Theut SK, Zaslow MJ, Rabinovich BA, Bartko JJ, Morihisa JM (1990). Resolution of parental bereavement after a perinatal loss. *J. Am. Acad. Child Adolesc. Psychiatry*, 29: 521–5.

Thorne SE (1993). *Negotiating Health Care: The Social Context of Chronic Illness*. Newbery Park, California: Sage.

Totman RG, Kiff J (1979). Life stress and susceptibility to colds. In DJ Oborne, MM Gruneberg and JR Eiser (Eds) *Research in Psychology and Medicine* Vol. I. London: Academic.

Townsend MB (1991). Creating a better work environment: Measuring effectiveness. *J. Nurs. Admin.*, 21: 11–4.

Tse K, Temple IK, Baraitser M (1990). Dilemmas in counselling: The EEC syndrome. *J. Med. Genet.*, 27: 752–5.

Tsunematsu Y (1988). Creation of a nursing environment with unrestricted communication among the staff: progress toward establishment of a conference system. *Nasu Suteshon*, 18: 31–6.

Tulving E (1972). Episodic and semantic memory. In E Tulving and WA Donaldson (Eds) *Organization of Memory*. New York: Academic Press.

Turk DC, Fernandez E (1990). On the putative uniqueness of cancer pain: Do psychological principles apply? *Beh. Res. Ther.*, 28: 1–13.

Turnbull F (1979). The nature of pain that may accompany cancer of the lung. *Pain*, 7: 371–5.

Twaddle AC (1981). Sickness and the sickness career: some implications. In L Eisenberg and A Klienman (Eds) *The Relevance of Social Science for Medicine*. Dordrecht: Elsevier.

Tyson J, Lasky R, Weiner M, Caldwell T, Sumner J (1984). Effect of nursing-staff support groups on the quality of newborn intensive care. *Crit. Care Med.*, 12: 901–6.

Ungar L, Florian V, Zernitski-Shurka E (1990). Aspects of fear of personal death, levels of awareness, and professional affiliation among dialysis unit staff members. *Omega*, 21: 51–67.

Vaillant EG (1976). Natural history of male psychological health. V. The relation of choice of ego mechanisms of defence to adult adjustment. *Arch. Gen. Psychiat.*, 33: 535–45.

Valman HM (1981). The handicapped child. *B.M.J.*, 283: 1166–9.

Van Eys J (1981). The truly cured child: the realistic and necessary goal in paediatric oncology. In JJ Spinetta and P Deasy-Spinetta (Eds) *Living With Childhood Cancer*. St. Louis: Moseby.

Van Wijk MG, Smalhout B (1990). A postoperative analysis of the patient's view of anaesthesia in a Netherlands' teaching hospital. *Anaesthesia*, 54: 679–82.

Vetter H, Ramsay LE, Luscher TF, Schrey A, Vetter W (1985). Symposium on compliance — Improving strategies in hypertension. *J. Hypertens.* (Supp.), 3: 1–99.

Videka-Sherman L (1982). Coping with the death of a child: A study over time. *Am. J. Orthopsychiat.*, 52: 688–98.

Viney LK, Henry R, Walker BM, Crooks L (1989). The emotional reactions of HIV antibody positive men. *Br. J. Med. Psychol.*, 62: 153–61.

Waechter EH (1987). The adolescent with Life-threatening chronic illness. In T. Krulik et al ibid.

Waechter E.H. (1987). Children's awareness of fatal illness. In T Krulik, B Holaday and IM Martinson (Eds) *The Child and Family Facing Life-threatening Illness.* Philadelphia: J.B. Lippincott Co.

Walsh S, Kinston RD (1988). The use of hospital beds for terminally ill cancer patients. *Eur. J. Surg. Oncol.*, 14: 367–70.

Walton J, McLachlan G (Eds) (1986). *Partnership or Prejudice: Communication Between Doctors and Those in the Other Caring Professions.* London: Nuffield Provincial Hospitals Trust.

Ward JD, Peat C, Revill J (1994) Deterioration in the N.H.S. (letter). *B.M.J.*, 308: 1239–40.

Wass H (1984). Parents, Teachers and Health Professionals as Helpers. In H Wass and CA Corr (Eds) *Helping Children Cope With Death: Guidelines and Resources* (2nd Ed). New York: Hemisphere Publishing Corp.

Weeks LC, Barrett M, Snead C (1985). Primary nursing. Teamwork is the answer. *J. Nurs. Adm.*, 15: 21–6.

Weiner S, Nathanson M (1976). Physical examination: Frequently observed errors. *J. Am. Med. Assoc.*, 236: 852–5.

Weiss L, Frischer L, Richman J (1989). Parental adjustment to intrapartum and delivery room loss. The role of a hospital-based support program. *Clin-Perinatol.*, 16: 1009–19.

Wellisch DK (1981). Intervention with the cancer patient. In CK Prokop and LA Bradley (Eds) *Medical Psychology: Contributions to Behavioural Medicine.* New York: Academic Press.

Wells KB, Benson C, Hoff P (1985). A model for teaching the brief psychosocial interview. *J. Med. Ed.*, 60: 181–8.

Whimster WF (1986). Communication between doctors and hospital laboratory staff. In J Walton and G. McLachlan (Eds) *Partnership or Prejudice: Communication Between Doctors and Those in the Other Caring Professions.* London: Nuffield Provincial Hospitals Trust.

Whiten A (Ed) (1991). *Natural Theories of Mind, Evolution, Development and Simulation.* Oxford: Blackwell.

Wild AA, Evans SJ (1968). The patient and the X-ray Department. *B.M.J.*, 270: 607–9.

Williams JMG, Watts FN, McLeod C, Mathews A (1988). *Cognitive Psychology and Emotional Disorders*. Chichester: Wiley.

Willis DJ, Elliot CH, Jay S (1982). Psychological effects of physical illness and its concomitants. In JM Tuna (Ed) *Handbook for the Practice of Paediatric Psychology*. New York: Wiley.

Wilkinson SR (1988). *The Child's World of Illness*. Cambridge: Cambridge University Press.

Woodforde JM, Fielding JR (1970). Pain and cancer. *J. Psychosomat. Res.*, 14: 365–70.

Woon TH (1983). Management of psychosocial aspects of children with cancer. *Postgraduate Doctor-Asia*, January: 13–5.

Wrate RM (1989). Talking to adolescents. In PR Myesrcough (Ed) *Talking With Patients. A Basic Clinical Skill*. Oxford: Oxford University Press.

Wright B (1990). A radiological presentation of neonatal and infantile syndromes. *Radiography Today*, 56: 17–20.

Youll JW (1989). The bridge beyond: strengthening nursing practice in attitudes towards death, dying and the terminally ill, and helping the spouses of critically ill patients. *Intensive Care Nurs.*, 5: 88–9.

Zajonc RB (1984). On the primacy of emotion. *American Psychologist*, 39: 117–23.

Zeanah CH (1989). Adaptation following perinatal loss: a critical review. *J. Am. Acad. Child. Adolesc. Psychiatry*, 28: 467–80.

Zbroski M (1969). *People in Pain*. San Francisco: Jossey-Bass.

Zweibel NR (1988). Measuring quality of life near the end of life. *J.A.M.A.*, 260: 839–40.

Index